T0220916

Interceptive
Orthodontics

A Practical Guide to Occlusal Management

To my family for their patience and support while I prepared this book, to the many postgraduate students I have had the pleasure of training and supervising for providing the inspiration for this book and to the patients who I hope have benefitted from the concepts behind this book.

Interceptive Orthodontics

A Practical Guide to Occlusal Management

Joseph Noar

MSc, BDS, FDSRCS(Ed), FDSRCS(Eng), DOrthRCS(Eng), MOrthRCS(Eng), FHEA

Consultant and Honorary Senior Lecturer
Orthodontic Unit
Division of Craniofacial & Development Sciences
Eastman Dental Hospital/Institute
London
UK

WILEY Blackwell

Library of Congress Cataloging-in-Publication Data

Noar, Joseph, author.
Interceptive orthodontics : a practical guide to occlusal management / Joseph Noar.
1 online resource.
Includes bibliographical references and index.
Description based on print version record and CIP data provided by publisher; resource not viewed.
ISBN 978-1-118-88027-2 (Adobe PDF) – ISBN 978-1-118-88028-9 (ePub) –
ISBN 978-0-470-65621-1 (pbk.)
I. Title.
[DNLM: 1. Malocclusion–therapy. 2. Maxillofacial Development. 3. Orthodontics, Corrective–methods. 4. Tooth–growth & development. WU 440]
RK527.5
617.6'43–dc23

2014021386

A catalogue record for this book is available from the British Library.

Wiley also publishes its books in a variety of electronic formats. Some content that appears in print may not be available in electronic books.

Cover images: courtesy of Joseph Noar

Set in 11/13 pt MeridienLTStd by Toppan Best-set Premedia Limited, Hong Kong

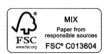

Contents

Preface, vii

1 Introduction, 1
What do we know about growth?, 1
Growth and development of the jaws, 2

2 Recognising the problem, 9
Is an attractive smile important?, 9

3 Investigations, 15
Radiographs, 15
Cone-beam computed tomography, 17
Study models, 23
Photographs, 24
What is the scope of orthodontic change?, 24

4 Managing the developing occlusion, 29
Thumb/finger sucking, 29
Crowding of the permanent lateral
incisors, 32

Serial extraction: a modern approach, 39
The unerupted central incisor, 42
Submerging deciduous second molars, 45
Fusion, gemination and morphology
issues, 47
Upper labial fraenum, 48
Leeway space and the use of intraoral
anchorage arches, 50
Sagittal problems: Class II, 51
Sagittal problems: Class III, 59
Ectopic and impacted teeth, 62
Missing teeth, 65

Index, 75

Preface

This book is aimed at the general dental practitioner, orthodontic trainee as well as specialist orthodontist. It covers the early stages of the development of the permanent dentition and aims to guide the practitioner in the practice of interceptive management of the developing dentition. The aim of this interceptive treatment is to promote the establishment of the permanent dentition within the line of the dental arches. This book addresses the issues of early crowding, impaction, supernumerary and supplemental teeth, dental arch expansion, space maintenance and space management. It will not only review the available evidence, but also provide clear treatment objectives and detailed treatment planning advice.

Joseph Noar
London, 2014

CHAPTER 1
Introduction

An attractive smile with a good display of teeth is important for psychological well-being. There are a number of goals that should be aimed for when considering dental attractiveness, such as the symmetry, alignment, smile line, dental arch shape and gingival contour, as well as the quality and morphology of the dental tissue itself. Orthodontic management of the developing dentition is important to ensure that the established dentition will be in the most aesthetic position. Orthodontics requires a good understanding of facial and dental growth and the effects of occlusal guidance.

In the past it was common practice for patients to be referred to an orthodontist once their secondary dentition was established. This practice allowed many developing problems to significantly worsen and ultimately be more difficult to correct. In many cases, developmental problems can be managed as the dentition develops and early intervention can eliminate some of the complex occlusal problems that can take 24 months or longer to manage with orthodontic appliances.

The premise of early interceptive treatment is to allow the secondary dentition to establish itself in an aesthetic position with the dental units lying within the dental arches. Issues such as skeletal discrepancy are managed within the scope of the genetic potential of each patient and early intervention should be decided on not only with reference to the severity of the discrepancy, but also the aesthetic and emotional needs of the patient and the implications of not undertaking treatment. For these reasons, general dental practitioners (GDPs) must consider early referral to a specialist orthodontist for all patients to ensure that all opportunities for occlusal guidance are taken. Referral at the age of 7 years allows any developing issues to be addressed in a strategic and planned manner.

What do we know about growth?

While a patient is still growing, there exists the possibility of addressing orthodontic problems with orthodontic appliances to alter facial growth. However, the problem in clinical orthodontics is that facial growth continues from birth to early adulthood and the growth pattern cannot be accurately predicted. We do know the average rate and direction of growth, but are aware of different skeletal relationships in three planes of space and of growth rotations that lead to differences in facial form from Class II to Class III, high and low angle and transverse discrepancies. We also have some understanding of the role of the facial

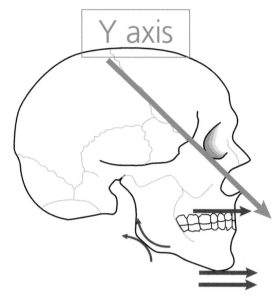

Figure 1.1 Directions of facial growth.

muscles and the influence environmental factors have on the dentition (Figure 1.1). However, we cannot reliably predict the timing of growth or the ultimate amount of growth for any individual until it is almost at an end, even if analytical techniques such as cervical spine and hand/wrist radiograph assessments are employed. In addition, while the soft tissue balance between the tongue, lips and cheeks and how this affects tooth position and dental arch shape can be predicted, we cannot quantify the latter over time or predict accurately the influences that these may have on the dental arch.

Growth and development of the jaws
Growth generally refers to an increase in size, number or complexity by natural development. Development is an increase in the degree of organisation (Proffit, 1993). Craniofacial growth may be divided into four components (Thilander, 1995):

1. growth mechanisms (how new bone is formed);

2. growth pattern (change in size and shape of the bone);
3. growth rate (speed at which the bone is formed);
4. regulating mechanism that initiates and directs the above three factors.

Growth mechanisms
Growth and development of the craniofacial skeleton occurs in two ways:
1. endochondral ossification: growth and ossification of a cartilage model;
2. intramembranous ossification: transformation of mesenchymal connective tissue and deposition of bone on existing bone surfaces.

The bones of the skull base mainly grow and develop by endochondral ossification, and the vault of the cranium and facial skeleton mainly by intramembranous ossification (Enlow, 1990).

Although several ossified areas fuse into large morphological units, remnants of the chondrocranium persist as synchondroses (cartilaginous joints) between the bones in the cranial base. When intramembranously formed bones meet, sutures develop. Bone growth and adaptation can thus proceed due to the separation of bones in the synchondroses and suture areas.

Growth of the cranial base
Displacement growth of the cranial base is made possible mainly by synchondroses. The spheno-occipital synchondrosis is regarded as the most important growth centre for the cranial base (Sicher, 1952; Björk, 1955). The upper facial skeleton is attached to the anterior cranial base, whereas the mandible is connected to the middle cranial base; thus, the length and growth of the cranial base has an important effect on the jaw relationships (Björk, 1955).

Growth of the mid-face

Scott (1953) suggested that the essential primary elements directing craniofacial skeletal growth are the cartilages, in particular the anterior extension of the chondrocranium, the nasal septal cartilage. The anteroposterior expansive growth of the nasal septal cartilage, which is buttressed against the cranial base posteriorly, is thought to 'push' the mid-face downward and forward and as such, the nasal septum is thought to play an important part in the prenatal and very early postnatal growth of the mid-face. However, opinions differ as to its role in postnatal growth; one view is that growth is secondary to, and compensatory for, passive displacement of the mid-facial bones and the nasal septum plays a significant biomechanical role in maintaining normal mid-facial form (Melsen, 1977; Moss, 1977).

Growth of the mandible

The cartilage of the mandibular condyle is a secondary cartilage and is different in origin and structure from the epiphyseal plate and synchondrosal cartilage (Thilander *et al.*, 1976).

The traditional view of the condylar cartilage was that it controlled overall mandibular growth and represented a major growth centre for the entire mandible (Scott, 1962). Koski and Makinen (1963) and Koski and Mason (1964) attempted to grow the condylar cartilages of rats and showed that cartilage only grew when it was explanted with the adjacent bone. Koski and his team interpreted this as confirmation of the views of Moss (1968) that growth of the condylar cartilage is always secondary to forward displacement of the mandible as a result of some outside influence, 'the functional matrix', and only participates in regional adaptive growth. They

suggested therefore, that condylar cartilage is not a major growth centre for the mandible, but it does have a great capacity to adapt to mandibular displacement during growth (Koski and Ronning, 1966; Enlow, 1990).

Experimental studies in animals by McNamara *et al.* (1982) have shown that cellular proliferation in the condylar cartilage can be influenced by appliances that displace the jaw forwards. However, the extent to which condylar growth can be modified in amount or direction by external influences is not clear. Displacement growth is made possible by the craniofacial sutures, which have the dual function of permitting growth movement and uniting the bones of the upper facial skeleton (Thilander, 1995). According to the Sutural Theory of Weinmann and Sicher (1947), the intrinsic pattern of expansive proliferative growth in the sutures generates forces that separate the bones and are thus responsible for the displacement of the maxillary complex. When sutures are transplanted to non-functional sites, however, no growth occurs (Ryoppy, 1965). Similarly, it has been demonstrated that growth of the circumaxillary sutures can be reduced or inhibited by the application of force to the maxilla (Elder and Tuenge, 1974). It is now accepted that facial sutures are not centres of active growth, but sites at which adaptive growth can occur in response to environmental demands (Moss and Salentijn, 1969).

All inner and outer bone surfaces of the facial skeleton are associated with a mosaic of functional growth fields. These fields carry out specific, localised growth activities that involve separate areas of resorption and deposition on all periosteal and endosteal surfaces (Enlow, 1990). Growth remodelling by periosteal resorption and deposition is paced by the growth and functions of the soft tissues in which the bones are embedded (Enlow, 1990). The influence of the periosteum is therefore of greatest significance with respect to the change in size and shape of the bones, i.e. the growth pattern (Enlow and Bang, 1965). The periosteum continues to function as an osteogenic zone throughout life, but its regenerative capacity is extremely high in the young child (Thilander, 1995).

Growth pattern

At birth the face makes up approximately one-eighth of the total volume of the skull, this proportion increasing to one-half in the adult male (Mills, 1983). The change in the size and shape of the bone takes place on the basis of several basic principles: remodelling, cortical drift, relocation, displacement and the 'V' principle (Enlow, 1990). These principles of bone growth will result in the following changes in size and shape of the nasomaxillary complex and the mandible.

Growth of the nasomaxillary complex

The postnatal growth of the maxillary complex occurs by sutural apposition and surface remodelling (Enlow and Bang, 1965).

The predominant direction of growth of the maxillary complex is posteriorly, with displacement occurring in the opposite anterior direction. As the growing maxillary complex is displaced, anteroposterior dimensions increase mainly by bone deposition on the tuberosity (Enlow, 1990). Simultaneously, the zygomatic region is relocated in a posterior direction (Enlow and Bang, 1965).

Vertical growth of the nasomaxillary complex, similar to the horizontal elongation, is brought about by a combination of growth remodelling and displacement associated with growth at the various sutures of the maxilla (Björk and Skieller, 1977). The palate is relocated inferiorly by a combination of periosteal resorption on the nasal side of the palate and periosteal deposition on the oral side. Simultaneously, periosteal resorption occurs on the anterior surface of the maxilla (Enlow and Bang, 1965).

Growth of the mandible

The postnatal growth of the mandible involves periosteal deposition at many sites. Elongation is brought about by deposition at the condyle and the posterior border of the ramus. Growth remodelling serves to maintain the shape and proportions of the bone as it increases in size (Enlow and Harris, 1964).

Displacement of the mandible is associated with a rotation dependent on the direction of condylar growth. Anterior rotation will take place in individuals with an upward and forward direction of condylar growth, whereas in those with a predominantly backward direction of condylar growth, the mandible will rotate in a posterior direction (Björk and Skieller, 1983).

The rate and direction of condylar growth is a secondary adaptive response to intrinsic and extrinsic biomechanical forces (Enlow, 1990). However, it is debateable whether it can be permanently changed by external forces acting only for a short time.

Growth rate

Craniofacial growth and development is a complex process that is not merely an increase in size; rather it is a differential growth process in which the various structures grow at different rates from birth to maturity (Enlow, 1966). Cross-sectional studies have identified differences in the growth curves of lymphoid, genital, neural and somatic tissues (Scammon, 1930). Growth of the calvarium follows the neural growth curve and reaches a plateau after 6 years of age. Growth of the facial skeleton follows the somatic growth curve and thus still has growth potential after the age of 6 years.

Although somatic tissues increase in size throughout the growth period, their growth rate is characterised by a decrease from birth with a minor mid-growth spurt at approximately 6–8 years of age, a prepubertal minimum, and a pubertal growth spurt (Brown *et al.*, 1970). The sequence of growth events is predictable, but their timing is quite variable among individuals. The developmental status of a child can be assessed by peak growth velocity in standing height, dental development, skeletal ossification and secondary sex characteristics (Moore *et al.*, 1990). Skeletal age, estimated from hand and wrist radiographs, has proved to be useful in helping to predict adult stature, but does not reliably predict the growth spurt (Houston, 1980). Menarche in girls and voice changes in boys occur soon after the peak of the growth spurt and so these features can be used to indicate whether or not the peak has passed (Hagg and Taranger, 1980). However, these assessments often can only report that growth has peaked and cannot be used to predict when it will peak if this has not occurred.

Growth in stature follows the somatic growth curve and has been investigated more thoroughly than has growth in facial dimensions, but it is a poor indicator of jaw growth (Houston *et al.*, 1997). The peak height velocity (pubertal growth spurt) was found by Tanner *et al.* (1976) to occur on average at 12 years of age in girls and at 14

years in boys, although they found considerable individual variation with a standard deviation of nearly 1 year.

Growth regulating mechanism
The control of a complex morphogenesis requires a precise biological regulatory mechanism for initiating and directing the growth mechanisms, growth pattern and growth rate (Thilander, 1995).

Sicher (1952) postulated that craniofacial growth as a whole was determined by the innate genetic information in the skeletal tissues; Scott (1962) postulated the heredity and expansive growth of the osteogenic tissues to the chondral structures; and Moss and Salentijn (1969) described the functional matrix theory, which refers to all the soft tissues and spaces that perform a given function such as mastication, swallowing and respiration, as being the stimulus for craniofacial skeletal growth.

Petrovic *et al.* (1990) carried out experimental work that led to the development of a cybernetic model of growth regulation, which states that it is the interaction of a series of causal changes and feedback mechanisms that determines the growth of the various parts of the craniofacial complex.

Craniofacial morphogenesis is now considered to be multifactorial, with facial development being influenced by several genes together with various environmental factors (Thilander, 1995). Van Limborgh (1982) has divided the factors controlling skeletal morphogenesis into five groups; namely, intrinsic genetic factors, local and general epigenetic factors, and local and general environmental influences. Essentially, growth is mainly under the influence of genetic factors rather than environmental ones (Figure 1.2).

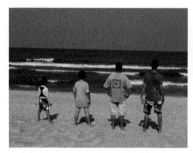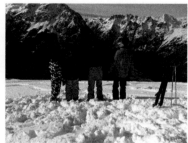

Figure 1.2 Growth is genetically controlled and largely not under our influence.

References

Björk A. (1955) Cranial base development. Am J Orthod. 41: 198–225.

Björk A, Skieller V. (1977) Growth of the maxilla in three dimensions as revealed radiographically by the implant method. Br J Orthod. 4: 53–64.

Björk A, Skieller V. (1983) Normal and abnormal growth of the mandible. A synthesis of longitudinal cephalometric implant studies over a period of 25 years. Eur J Orthod. 5: 1–46

Brown T, Barrett MJ, Grave KC. (1970) Facial growth and skeletal maturation at adolescence. Tandlaegebladet. 75: 1221–1222. Cited by Moore RN, Moyer BA, DuBois LM. (1990) Skeletal maturation and craniofacial growth. Am J Orthod Dentofacial Orthop. 98: 33–40.

Elder JR, Tuenge RH. (1974) Cephalometric and histologic changes produced by extraoral high-pull traction to the maxilla in *Macaca mulatta*. Am J Orthod. 66: 599–617.

Enlow DH. (1966) A morphogenetic analysis of facial growth. Am J Orthod. 52: 283–299.

Enlow DH. (1990) Facial Growth, 3rd edn. W.B. Saunders Co., Philadelphia.

Enlow DH, Bang S. (1965) Growth and remodeling of the human maxilla. Am J Orthod. 51: 446.

Enlow DH, Harris DB. (1964) A study of the postnatal growth of the human mandible. Am J Orthod. 50: 25–50.

Hagg U, Taranger J. (1980) Menarche and voice change as indicators of the pubertal growth spurt. Acta Odontol Scand. 38: 179–186.

Houston WJ. (1980) Relationships between skeletal maturity estimated from hand-wrist radiographs and the timing of the adolescent growth spurt. Eur J Orthod. 2: 81–93.

Houston WJB, Stephens CD, Tulley WJ. (1997) A Textbook of Orthodontics, 2nd rev. edn. Wright Co., Oxford.

Koski K, Makinen L. (1963) Growth potential of transplanted components of the mandibular ramus. I. Suom Hammaslaak Toim. 59: 296–308. Cited by Mills JR. (1983) A clinician looks at facial growth. Br J Orthod. 10: 58–72.

Koski K, Mason KE. (1964) Growth potential of transplanted components of the mandibular ramus. II. Suom Hammaslaak Toim. 60: 209–219. Cited by Mills JR. (1983) A clinician looks at facial growth. Br J Orthod. 10: 58–72.

Koski K, Ronning O. (1966) Growth potential of transplanted components of the mandibular ramus. III. Suom Hammaslaak Toim. 61: 291–297. Cited by Mills JR. (1983) A clinician looks at facial growth. Br J Orthod. 10: 58–72.

McNamara JA, Jr, Hinton RJ, Hoffman DL. (1982) Histologic analysis of temporomandibular joint adaptation to protrusive function in young adult rhesus monkeys (Macaca mulatta). Am J Orthod. 82: 288–298.

Melsen, B. (1977) Histological analysis of the postnatal development of the nasal septum. Angle Orthod. 47: 83–96.

Mills JRE. (1983) A clinician looks at facial growth. Br J Orthod. 10: 58–72.

Moore RN, Moyer BA, DuBois LM. (1990) Skeletal maturation and craniofacial growth. Am J Orthod Dentofacial Orthop. 98: 33–40.

Moss ML. (1968) The primacy of functional matrices in orofacial growth. Dent Pract Dent Rec. 19: 65–73.

Moss ML. (1977) The role of the nasal septal cartilage in midfacial growth. In: McNamara JA Jr, ed. Factors Affecting Growth of the Midface. Monograph 6, Craniofacial Growth Series. Needham Press, Ann Arbor, MI.

Moss ML, Salentijn L. (1969) The primary role of functional matrices in facial growth. Am J Orthod. 55: 566–577.

Petrovic AG, Stutzmann JJ, Lavergne JM. (1990) Mechanisms of craniofacial growth and modus operandi of functional appliances: a cell level and cybernetic approach to orthodontic decision making. In: Carlson DS, ed. Craniofacial Growth Theories and Orthodontic Treatment. Monograph 23. Craniofacial Growth Series, Needham Press, Ann Arbor, MI.

Proffit WR. (1993) Contemporary Orthodontics, 2nd edn. Mosby-Year Book, Inc., St. Louis.

Ryoppy S. (1965) Transplantation of epiphyseal cartilage and cranial suture. Experimental studies on the preservation of the growth capacity in growing bone grafts. Acta Orthop Scand. Suppl: 1–106.

Scammon RE. (1930) The measurement of the body in childhood. In: Harris JA, Jackson CM, Paterson DG, Scammon RE. The Measurement of Man. University of Minnesota Press, Minneapolis, MN.

Scott JH. (1953) The cartilage of the nasal septum. Br J Orthod. 95: 37–43.

Scott JH. (1962) The growth of the craniofacial skeleton. Int J Med Sci. 438: 276–286.

Sicher H. (1952) Oral Anatomy. CV Mosby Co., St. Louis.

Tanner JM, Whitehouse RH, Marubini E, Resele LF. (1976) The adolescent growth spurt of boys and girls of the Harpenden growth study. Ann Hum Biol. 3: 109–126.

Thilander B. (1995) Basic mechanisms in craniofacial growth. Acta Odontol Scand. 53(3): 144–151.

Thilander B, Carlsson GE, Ingervall B. (1976) Postnatal development of the human temporomandibular joint. I. A histological study. Acta Odontol Scand. 34: 117–126.

van Limborgh J. (1982) Factors controlling skeletal morphogenesis. Prog Clin Biol Res. 101: 1–17.

Weinmann JP, Sicher H. (1947) Bone and Bones. Fundamentals of bone biology. CV Mosby Co., St. Louis.

CHAPTER 2
Recognising the problem

Is an attractive smile important?

Facial attractiveness impacts on how an individual is seen by others, and a good display of well-aligned teeth is important for psychological well-being. The smile line is important; the incisal edges of the upper incisors should follow the lower lip, with almost the full crown displayed to give good facial balance. In addition, the dental arch should be broad with the first and perhaps the second premolars showing.

Specific angles or measurements cannot be prescribed for facial aesthetics as we are all different, but in general good facial aesthetics is dictated by:
- symmetry;
- harmony;
- balance.

The overall facial attractiveness depends on the skeletal relationship of the maxilla and mandible, and the tone and movement of the soft tissues.

From a clinical perspective it is important to remember that the position of the teeth is reliant on the position of the jaws within the facial skeleton, the effects of the soft tissue forces of the tongue intraorally and the cheeks and lips extraorally, and the relative sizes of the jaws. It is also important to consider racial and sexual differences in the position of the dentition.

During the initial assessment of a patient it is important to have an overall impression of facial form and head posture. The facial form of the child is likely to be similar to that of other members of the family, so an assessment of siblings and both parents will be very helpful in determining the likely growth pattern of the child. A full medical and dental history should always be taken to highlight any factors that could impact on the growth or treatment of the child. The physical growth status of the child should be assessed to determine if their chronological and developmental ages are consistent. Clinical examination is everything (Figure 2.1).

Clinical assessment of the anteroposterior (A–P) plane is done by palpating for the clinical A point (the maximum concavity of the anterior part of the maxilla) and B point (the maximum concavity of the anterior part of the mandible) (Figure 2.2). This will give the rough position of the maxilla relative to the mandible. In a Class I relationship the maxilla is a few millimetres behind the mandible. With the fingers (either intra- or extra-orally) on the A and B points, the clinician can 'feel' if there is a discrepancy. Normally, the first finger is a few millimetres shorter than the middle finger. If the skeletal bases are basically Class I, the fingers will lie straight as the maxilla should be a few millimetres ahead of the mandible. If there is a significant discrepancy, one or other finger will be bent.

Interceptive Orthodontics: A Practical Guide to Occlusal Management, First Edition. Joseph Noar.
© 2014 John Wiley & Sons, Ltd. Published 2014 by John Wiley & Sons, Ltd.

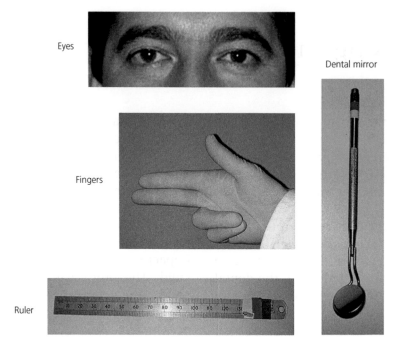

Eyes

Fingers

Ruler

Dental mirror

Figure 2.1 Essential clinical assessment tools.

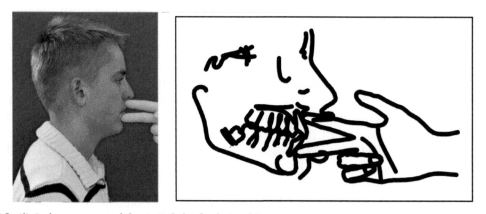

Figure 2.2 Clinical assessment of the A–P skeletal relationship.

The vertical plane is assessed by judging the angle of the mandible to the maxilla (MM angle) when the patient is sitting with the Frankfort plane parallel to the floor, and placing the finger and thumb on the jawline as shown in Figure 2.3. If the index finger points through the occiput, the MM angle is essentially normal. Vertical facial proportions are divided into thirds with the lower third (chin point to subna-

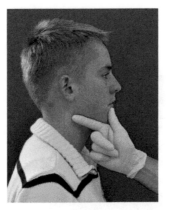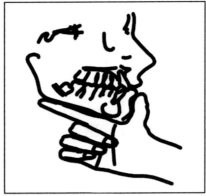

Figure 2.3 Clinical assessment of the maxillary mandibular angle.

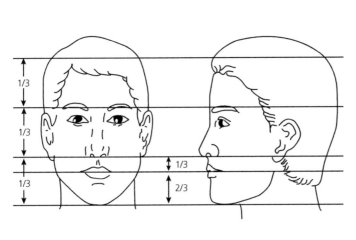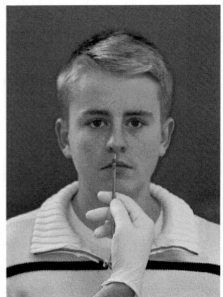

Figure 2.4 Clinical assessment of the lower anterior face height.

sale) equal to the mid third (subnasale to glabella) if the patient has average proportions (Figure 2.4).

For good aesthetics the face should be essentially symmetrical with the corners of the mouth the same width as the interpupillary distance, and the nasal alar cartilages in the same plane as the inner canthus of the eyes (Figure 2.5). Most individuals have mild transverse asymmetries and assessment is usually made from clinical judgement alone.

In the assessment of facial form it is important not to be caught out by dental displacements as these can produce a facial asymmetry due to the movement of the

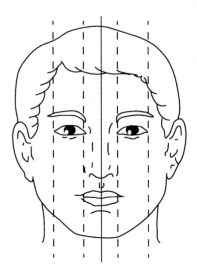 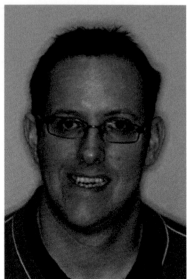

Figure 2.5 Clinical assessment of facial symmetry.

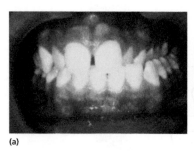 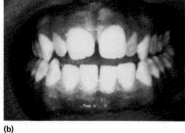

(a)   (b)

Figure 2.6 Facial asymmetry can be caused by mandibular displacement due to crossbites with displacements. (a) Displaced position; (b) first contact with condyles in retruded axis position.

mandible with respect to the maxilla. To avoid this possibility, always ensure that the mandible is assessed in the retruded contact position (Figure 2.6).

Overjet (OJ) and overbite (OB) are measured with an intraoral ruler. OJ is measured from the labial surface of the lower incisors to the incisal edge of the most prominent upper incisor (Figure 2.7). It is important to consider the relationship of the incisors to the lower lip and the inclination of the incisors in this assessment. The lower lip controls the position of the upper

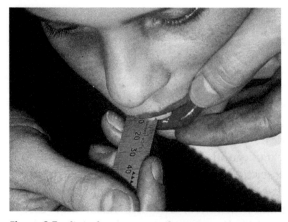

Figure 2.7 Clinical assessment of overjet.

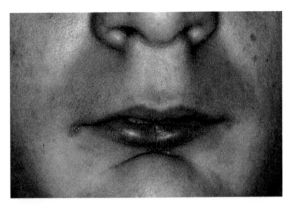

Figure 2.8 Lip trap (upper right incisor resting on lower lip).

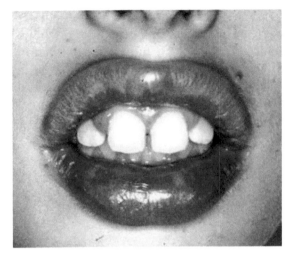

Figure 2.9 Lip apart posture at rest.

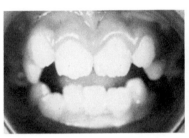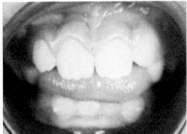

Figure 2.10 Forward tongue position causing an anterior open bite.

incisors and a lip trap can cause significant proclination of the teeth (Figure 2.8). If the lips are not together at rest and the lower lip lies below the incisal edge of the upper incisors, there is no control of their labial position (Figure 2.9).

If the OJ is increased, there is an increased risk of trauma (33% increased risk with an OJ of >6 mm and 40% with an OJ of >8 mm). If the OB is deep and complete to the palate, this can cause soft tissue damage. Although periodontists are clear that with excellent oral hygiene, palatal trauma from the lower incisors can be controlled without soft tissue damage, if the oral hygiene is poor or there is trauma to the palatal gingivae, the tissues can become inflamed. This can be exacerbated by the trauma of biting into the inflamed tissue and lead to further swelling and a spiral of damage that can cause permanent gingival loss. Even with excellent oral hygiene, during eating the tissues can be damaged by biting into something hard or sharp such that a deep bite is always a cause for concern in the long term.

Tongue thrusts are rare, but adaptive swallowing patterns with the tongue providing an anterior oral seal in those with anterior open bites is common (Figure 2.10).

It is also important in an orthodontic assessment to undertake a comprehensive dental examination to ensure there is no caries or periodontal disease, adequate levels of attached gingivae and no bone dehiscences that can impact on extraction choices and treatment planning. Plaque indexes are a good indicator of the oral hygiene status of the patient and enamel hypoplasias should be noted, particularly if fixed appliances are being considered. Temporomandibular joint (TMJ) function has been shown to be independent of orthodontic treatment, but should still be assessed to rule out any significant disease.

CHAPTER 3

Investigations

Radiographs

The orthopantogram (OPG) and anterior occlusal radiographs are the X-rays of choice for an orthodontic examination, and allow for the assessment of the presence of teeth, their position, the degree of crowding and any bone pathology, as well as the basic quality of the dentition and of restorations (Figure 3.1). Early assessment

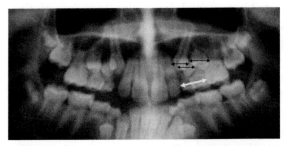

Figure 3.1 OPG radiograph: Simple assessment of the space requirements for the developing dentition.

is important as often ectopically positioned teeth or hypodontia can be managed by the early extraction of primary teeth. The position of the maxillary canines is particularly unpredictable and can be identified in three planes of space by using vertical parallax with OPG and upper anterior occlusal radiographs. Parallax employs the tube shift method of radiographic localisation of objects: an object that is near to the source of the X-rays will move in the opposite direction to the shift in the X-ray tube and those further away will move in the same direction. An OPG is fixed in the horizontal plane and the anterior occlusal radiograph is at roughly 60° to the horizontal and requires a 'shift' in the tube position. By comparing an unerupted tooth to the root of an adjacent tooth, its bucco-palatal position can be accurately determined (Figure 3.2).

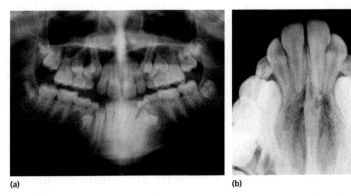

(a)   (b)

Figure 3.2 (a) OPG radiograph to identify maxillary canine position using vertical parallax. (b) Standard occlusal radiograph.

Interceptive Orthodontics: A Practical Guide to Occlusal Management, First Edition. Joseph Noar.
© 2014 John Wiley & Sons, Ltd. Published 2014 by John Wiley & Sons, Ltd.

Assessing crowding on OPG radiographs

This method of assessing crowding has the advantage of being able to predict at an early stage whether extractions will be necessary as part of comprehensive orthodontic treatment. Although there is often distortion on a tomograph, although the image of the posterior segments is usually easily visualised and gross measurements can be easily made. By measuring the mesio-distal widths of the canines and premolars and the distance between the distal edge of the lateral incisor and the mesial edge of the first molar, a reasonable assessment of the dento-alveolar disproportion can be made. Obviously, as the dentition erupts, there will be considerable further growth and development, but these measurements give a very good indication if extractions are necessary. Where there is significant crowding, early extraction of a premolar unit will allow space for the eruption of a canine and second premolar unit into the line of the dental arch without becoming ectopic. This will shorten the orthodontic treatment or even eliminate the need for it. If the crowding is assessed to be mild, the clinician will have additional justification for early arch expansion if there is an asymmetric maxillary arch or crossbite.

Cephalometric evaluation

A lateral cephalograph can be used to assess the jaw position, to monitor craniofacial growth and mandibular rotations, and to identify changes with treatment (Figure 3.2). Cephalometric evaluation provides numeric data to identify skeletal and dental discrepancies; however, it must be remembered that this evaluation only supports the clinical diagnosis and that numeric data do not always translate into good aesthetics. Great care has to be taken during treat-ment planning not to give undue importance to specific angles and distances measured on these radiographs, as overall facial aesthetics is the primary goal (Figure 3.3).

If a cephalometric assessment indicates the upper incisors are inclined beyond the expected normal value for that individual, this does not mean that the teeth are pro-clined in the face or that they are unstable. It is possible that the maxilla is positioned such that the incisors are aesthetically pleasing even at this increased angulation. However, treatment changes (the changes in tooth inclination with appliances) can be reasonably accurately assessed using measurements taken from a lateral cephalo-graph. The relationship of the skeletal bases can be assessed from the severity of the discrepancy between the upper and lower jaws. Once this has been determined, the amount of dento-alveolar change needed to satisfy the patient's wishes and to ensure reasonable post-treatment tooth position can be assessed. The stability of the tooth position after orthodontic treatment is uncertain and depends not only on growth but also on soft tissue balance as well as the initial tooth displacement. Current think-ing is that the stability of the tooth position cannot be guaranteed as the soft tissue 'neutral zone' in which the teeth sit (with the tongue pushing out and the lips and cheeks pushing in) together with the effect of the periodontal and supragingival fibres change with maturity. Whether the neutral zone is wide or narrow, it cannot be pre-dicted whether this width will change over time and therefore stability of individual teeth after orthodontic tooth movement can only be guaranteed by using retainers. The amount of time retainers need to be worn, both in terms of hours per day and for how many months or years, is always subjective and will be different for each

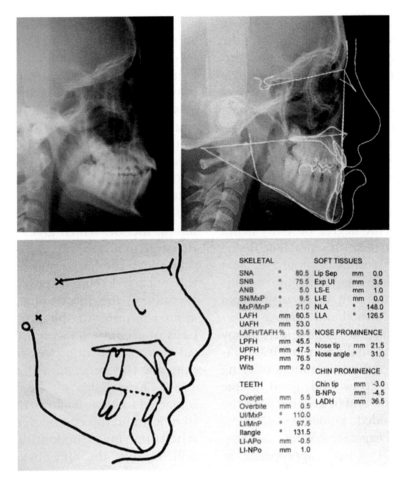

Figure 3.3 Lateral cephalograph and analysis.

individual patient. The decision must be made by considering both the initial malocclusion and the amount of tooth movement to be achieved during treatment. Cephalometric analysis should *never* be used to predict stability.

Cone-beam computed tomography

Cone-beam computed tomography (CBCT) is a fast developing technology that provides relatively low-dose, high spatial resolution imaging of the craniofacial complex in three dimensions (3D) (De Vos *et al.*, 2009). It is increasingly being utilised in orthodontics, oral and maxillofacial surgery, implantology and restorative dentistry. CBCT has proven especially useful for the location of pathology and delineation of structures, but care has to be taken as the detailed information gained from 3D imaging can expose our limitations in interpreting the findings. Identification of pathology that is not routinely seen on 2D images can lead to confusion or clinical error if clinicians are unable to interpret or manage the findings because of the limited evidence base.

CBCT utilises a cone-shaped X-ray beam, which rotates synchronously around the patient's head with an area detector. This captures an entire region of interest in a single rotation of the radiation source, unlike the 'multiple slices' that are generated by conventional CT (Kau *et al.*, 2005). CBCT output gives a cylindrically shaped volume of the patient's bony skeleton. The volumetric data set contained in this 'cylinder' consists of a 3D block of cuboid structures, known as voxels. Each voxel represents a specific degree of X-ray beam absorption. Image reconstruction is achieved using computer software programs that utilise sophisticated algorithms and reconstructing the images in three orthogonal planes; sagittal, coronal and axial.

CBCT is an effective imaging technology producing dimensionally accurate information, with small volume scanners offering lower radiation doses and good image quality. At present, and in keeping with the latest recommended guidelines (*Ionising Radiation Medical Exposure Regulations 2000*), the use of CBCT is only appropriate in select cases where conventional radiography has failed to provide adequate diagnostic information (Arai *et al.*, 1999). A number of areas where CBCT is useful are described here. Others that are outside the scope of this book include planning for temporary anchorage devices, rapid maxillary expansion, cleft palate and orthognathic surgery.

Detection of impacted/ectopic teeth

Current mainstream practice for the localisation of impacted teeth involves 2D radiographic imaging using conventional radiographs, such as dental panoramic tomograms (OPGs) and periapical views, which provide information about the vertical and mesio-distal relationships of the unerupted tooth with neighbouring teeth and roots. These radiographs may be supplemented with other 2D images, such as occlusal radiographs and lateral cephalograms. However, plain film 2D imaging may not be sufficient for the identification of structures because of distortion, magnification and imaging artefacts, particularly in the presence of superimpositions associated with adjacent structures (Bodner *et al.*, 2001). The 3D image sets provided by CBCT allow a more precise localisation of the impacted canine with respect to the lateral incisor, which gives the orthodontic surgeon a clear picture of what will be seen when the flap is raised at surgery and the impacted tooth exposed (Figure 3.4). Identifying the most appropriate surgical approach prior to the procedure on the basis of accurate imaging minimises surgical trauma and improves the periodontal outcome (Becker *et al.*, 1983; Kohavi *et al.*, 1984). Knowledge of the location of an impacted tooth also allows the orthodontist to determine the correct vector to be used when applying orthodontic traction, which will improve the efficiency of the orthodontic mechanics and minimise any unnecessary manipulation of the impacted tooth (Figure 3.5).

Detection of root resorption associated with impacted teeth

A fundamental component of diagnosis is not only the accurate location of an impacted tooth, but also the detection of any adjacent tooth root resorption (Figure 3.4). However, accurate information regarding the degree of external root resorption in itself does not provide an absolute guide to subsequent treatment planning decisions. Indeed, whilst the introduction of CBCT has facilitated the acquisition of information that can lead to improved rates of resorption detection (up to 50%) (Ericson

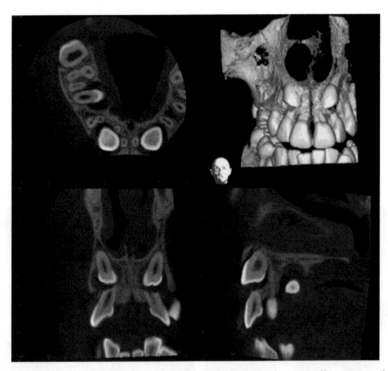

Figure 3.4 CBCT images in the X, Y and Z planes showing buccally placed ectopically positioned upper left and right canines overlying the roots of the upper lateral incisors. The images show significant resorption of the roots of these teeth and enlarged canine crown follicles. The reconstructed slices are also shown in 3D. Using these images it is possible to make a judgement in all planes as to the likely long-term prognosis for the lateral incisors. The difficulty at the present time is the lack of evidence for or understanding of what happens to the resorption once the canines have been moved away from the incisors. It is important within the treatment planning process to know if the resorption will continue or remain stable. These images demonstrate both the good visualisation of the area and our limitations in interpreting this information.

and Kurol, 2000; Gracco *et al.*, 2008; Alqerban *et al.*, 2009), there are currently no studies that have investigated the long-term course of this resorption or the effects of different treatment modalities, such as orthodontic traction to move the impacted tooth away from the affected root. Without this information, great care must be taken when formulating a treatment plan.

Detection of supernumerary teeth
(Figure 3.5b)
Impaction of maxillary incisors is frequently associated with the presence of unerupted supernumerary teeth. Localisation with 2D imaging, particularly with OPG, can be challenging, especially the determination of the labio-lingual order of the supernumerary teeth, their relative heights, the normality of their crowns and the root anatomy. If a patient is sent to a radiology department for their radiographs, it is not possible to control the angle at which intraoral views are taken and therefore errors of perspective cannot be ruled out. Without CBCT, a true picture of the arrangement of the supernumerary teeth can only be ascertained when a tooth is surgically exposed. In comparison, by providing detailed 3D information, CBCT can

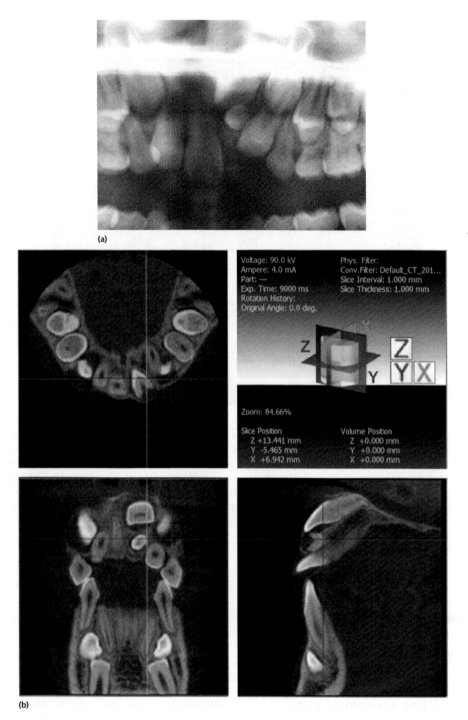

Figure 3.5 (a) Section from a DPT showing the presence of a supernumerary tooth associated with the upper left central incisor – the diagnostic information is limited, as accurate localisation is not possible. (b) CBCT images in the X, Y and Z planes showing the position in 3D of a supernumerary palatal to the ectopically positioned upper central incisor. These views provide excellent positional information for this tooth and the morphology of both its crown and root and the surrounding alveolar bone. This information is particularly important to the orthodontic surgeon as it allows removal with maximum accuracy and therefore minimal trauma. By assessing the orientation of the unerupted tooth, a view can be reached as to whether it will move away from the other teeth (and can therefore be left to be reviewed) or whether it is likely to be an obstruction that requires removal.

detail the morphology and relationship of a tooth to adjacent structures, including one-to-one measurements of distances, which allows for much better diagnostic accuracy. However, in order to reduce radiation exposure to the patient it is of course important to gain as much information as possible from existing plain film radiographs before recommending CBCT and then, only imaging the areas where pathology is suspected.

Detection of developmental anomalies

This is one situation where CBCT has significantly improved assessment and treatment planning. In order to align an incisor with a talon cusp and provide a functional and well interdigitated occlusion, the enamel extension often needs to be reduced. Prior to CBT it was not possible to determine how far the pulpal tissue extended into the cusp. CBCT is ideal for this purpose (Figure 3.6).

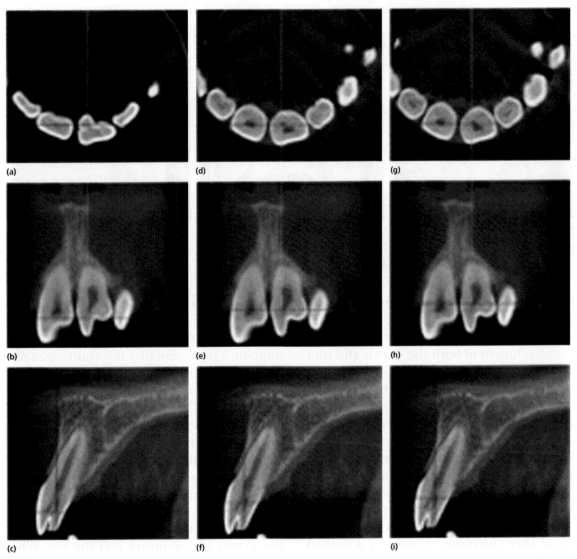

(a) (d) (g)

(b) (e) (h)

(c) (f) (i)

Figure 3.6 CBCT imaging at different heights showing the talon cusp and clearly demonstrating the degree of extension of pulpal tissue into the cusp.

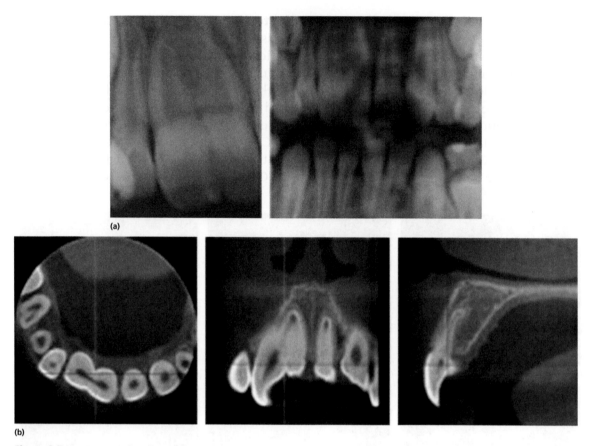

(a)

(b)

Figure 3.7 (a) Periapical radiograph (2D image) showing fusion of the incisor teeth. (b) CBCT image (3D) showing accurately the extent of root and crown contact.

In addition, CBCT can also provide useful information in the assessment of fused and geminated teeth, particularly the extent of the attachment of both the crown and root portions of these 'double' teeth. It can clearly show whether the tooth can be sectioned or not if there is too much attachment along the root length (Figure 3.7).

Detection of a root fracture

The management of a root fracture is difficult. It is very important to determine where the fracture line is in order to decide whether treatment to the proximal portion could save the tooth, if only for a limited period. In the younger patient, the preservation of alveolar bone by retaining either the proximal or distal part of the tooth or both is a great advantage if eventual implant replacement is contemplated. Careful assessment of the degree and position of root fractures can be clearly visualised with CBCT, as can the quality of any subsequent restoration, which is a great help in the treatment planning process (Figure 3.8). Two-dimensional analysis can demonstrate a fracture, but 3D CBCT can quantify it in all planes, exposing any 'shelving' fracture to its full extent and allowing a much clearer understanding of the extent of the injury and the possibilities for restoration.

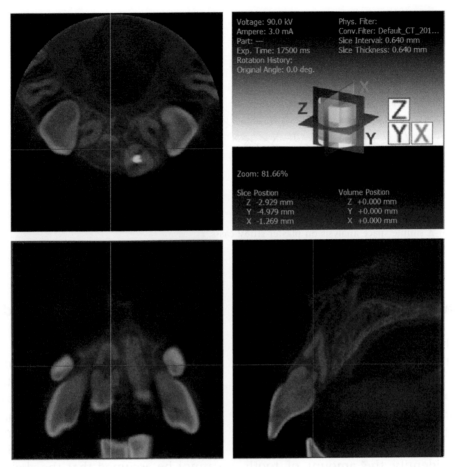

Figure 3.8 CBCT images in the X, Y and Z planes, allowing comprehensive analysis of the root fracture affecting the UR1. The level of the root fracture, any shelving and any microfractures can be visualised. This allows accurate treatment planning and assessment of any repair. Progressive resorption can also be monitored accurately.

Study models

Taking study casts is an invaluable way of viewing the whole of the occlusion, allowing assessment of dental relationships and an assessment of crowding within the arches as well as tooth inclination and overbite. Simple space analysis can be carried out by measuring the individual tooth mesio-distal widths of each tooth from second premolar to second premolar and the arch segments from the mesial of the first molar to the mesial of the first premolar and the distal edge of the canine to the mesial edge of the central incisor (Figure 3.9). By subtracting one from the other, an assessment of the tooth/arch discrepancy can be made.

The one great difficulty with study casts is that impressions must be taken to produce them. Many younger patients find this very unpleasant and for them digital photography or even digital scanning may be a better way of recording the dental position.

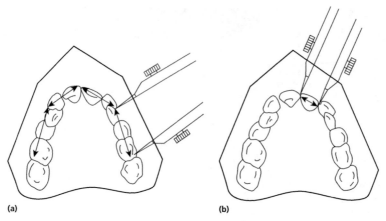

Figure 3.9 (a,b) A simple space analysis on plaster study casts.

Photographs

Photographs are an invaluable tool for the assessment of change in orthodontics (Figures 3.10 and 3.11). They should be taken to provide start and finish records and be used as a reference for growth and treatment progress. Extraoral views should be taken with the patient relaxed and smiling to identify the amount of tooth exposure and any abnormal lip morphology. As digital photography has advanced, it has become the clinical record of choice.

Photography is a very important part of orthodontic communication and is often very useful in patient education. Photographs can be used to motivate a patient and to demonstrate treatment changes. Photographs also can record any issues that could lead to conflict, such as enamel hypoplasia and white spots that were present before treatment. As it is common for patients to transfer their care if they move home or country, electronic transfer of information is easy and effective with digital photography.

What is the scope of orthodontic change?

There is a huge amount of evidence available regarding the scope of orthodontic change and to predict orthodontic changes, it is important to understand what orthodontic appliances can do (Proffit and White, 1990). From the available evidence it cannot be assumed that the skeletal bases will move substantially under the influence of orthodontic appliances. However, it must be assumed that the mandible will and can only grow to its full growth potential and that maxillary growth cannot be substantially changed. It may be possible to release a mandible that has been held back by environmental factors (soft tissues or dentition) or to encourage a mandible that is growing slowly to 'speed up'. It may even be possible to enhance the anterior development of the maxilla, but this change will be temporary and the skeletal pattern will return to its genetically programmed position once appliance wear has ceased. Dental movement within the bone and dento-

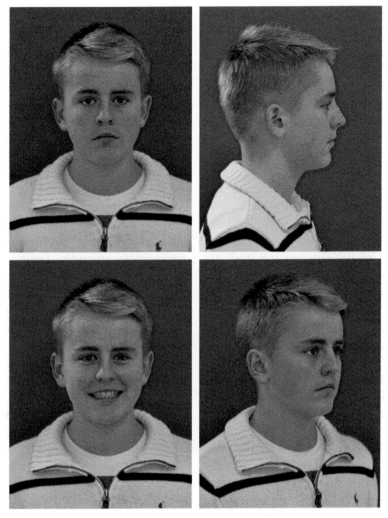

Figure 3.10 Extraoral photographs.

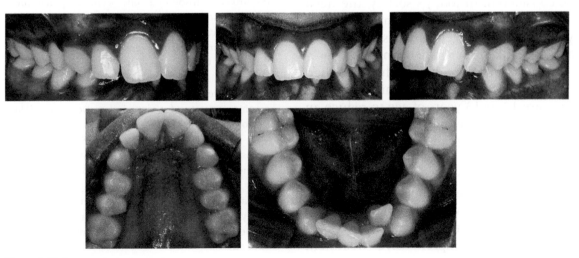

Figure 3.11 Intraoral photographs.

alveolar bending are possible, but will only be stable within the particular soft tissue and skeletal balance.

Before treatment, therefore, it must be decided how much change needs to be made and how severe the skeletal discrepancy is. It needs to be determined if dentoalveolar and dental movement alone can camouflage the problem and if the facial and dental aesthetics with camouflage alone can address the patient's concerns. In addition to these objectives, it is important to determine if the patient can (or wishes to) cooperate with treatment.

It is also current practice to delay treatment to be sure of the growth changes that may occur. This may not be the best approach as psychological factors and the needs of the patient may outweigh the disadvantages of early treatment. This is a fundamental issue in this book. If it is accepted that the amount of skeletal change is limited and the soft tissues are not under orthodontic control, then the timing of treatment is not bound to the pubertal growth spurt. Early treatment based on psychological and clinical need should drive the start of orthodontic treatment. The different reasons for undertaking orthodontic treatment should be considered. In today's society, the need for good dental aesthetics is apparent at a younger and younger age. Teasing at school and the risk of permanent injury to proclined incisors should be addressed when requested. Making a young child wait until they are 12 or 13 years of age to reduce an overjet or improve the position of crowded incisors is not acceptable. Children from the age of 7 years are quite capable of understanding and accepting orthodontic treatment. In fact, there is good reason to believe that compliance with treatment at 7–10 years of age is much more likely than at 11–14 years. Comprehensive treatment cannot be carried out until all the permanent teeth (with the exception of the third molars) are present, so treatment has to be specific, effective and appropriate to the child's needs and wishes without compromising later treatment. Interceptive guidance of the developing permanent teeth and early appliance therapy should be seen as part of the orthodontic journey for those who wish for it.

Why do some treatments work and others fail? This is usually down to lack of appropriate growth, poor clinical assessment, poor patient selection, poorly made appliances, poor patient motivation and incorrect instructions on how to wear the appliances. Patients who do well with orthodontic appliances are usually those with mild skeletal discrepancies, no abnormal soft tissue factors, and who are motivated and have a clear idea of what they want to be achieved. Patients who do less well often have severe skeletal discrepancies or are disinterested in the process.

References

Alqerban A, Jacobs R, Souza PC, Willems G. (2009) In-vitro comparison of 2 cone-beam computed tomography systems and panoramic imaging for detecting simulated canine impaction-induced external root resorption in maxillary lateral incisors. Am J Orthod Dentofacial Orthop. 136: 764–711.

Arai Y, Tammisalo E, Iwai K, Hashimoto K, Shinoda K. (1999) Development of a compact computed tomographic apparatus for dental use. Dentomaxillofac Radiol. 28: 245–248.

Becker A, Kohavi D, Zilberman Y. (1983) Periodontal status following the alignment of palatally impacted canine teeth. Am J Orthod. 84: 332–336.

Bodner L, Bar-Ziv J, Becker A. (2001) Image accuracy of plain film radiography and computerized tomography in assessing morphological abnormality of impacted teeth. Am J Orthod Dentofacial Orthop. 120: 623–628.

De Vos W, Casselman J, Swennen GR. (2009) Cone-beam computerized tomography (CBCT) imaging of the oral and maxillofacial region: a systematic review of the literature. Int J Oral Maxillofac Surg. 38: 609–625.

Ericson S, Kurol PJ. (2000) Resorption of incisors after ectopic eruption of maxillary canines: a CT study. Angle Orthod. 70: 415–423.

Gracco A, Lombardo L, Cozzani M, Siciliani G. (2008) Quantitative cone-beam computed tomography evaluation of palatal bone thickness for orthodontic miniscrew placement. Am J Orthod Dentofacial Orthop. 134: 361–369.

Kau CH, Richmond S, Palomo JM, Hans MG. (2005) Three-dimensional cone beam computerized tomography in orthodontics. J Orthod. 32: 282–293.

Kohavi D, Becker A, Zilberman Y. (1984) Surgical exposure, orthodontic movement, and final tooth position as factors in periodontal breakdown of treated palatally impacted canines. Am J Orthod. 85: 72–77.

Proffit WR, White RP. (1990) Who needs surgical-orthodontic treatment? Int J Adult Orthognath Surg 5: 81–89.

CHAPTER 4
Managing the developing occlusion

Thumb/finger sucking

Thumb/finger sucking can cause significant distortion of the dental arches. The severity of this is related to the amount of time spent digit sucking each day and the method and intensity with which the individual sucks (Warren *et al.*, 2005). It has been reported that up to 70% of 10-year olds have a digit sucking habit and that two-thirds of these can end up with a serious malocclusion as a result. Studies have shown that the main effects of a persistent habit can include a reduced overbite or mild anterior open bite, and a mild tendency to proclination of the upper incisors with tendency to mild posterior crossbites as a result of the negative pressure produced by the sucking. More serious effects, such as an asymmetric open bite or severe posterior crossbites are much rarer (Figures 4.1 and 4.2) (Popovich, 1966; Mitchell,

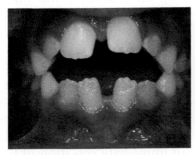
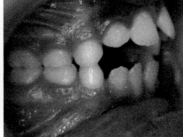

Figure 4.1 Effect of thumb sucking on the dentition.

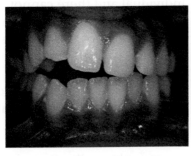
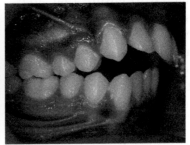

Figure 4.2 Asymmetric open bite due to digit sucking.

Interceptive Orthodontics: A Practical Guide to Occlusal Management, First Edition. Joseph Noar.
© 2014 John Wiley & Sons, Ltd. Published 2014 by John Wiley & Sons, Ltd.

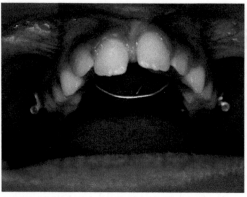 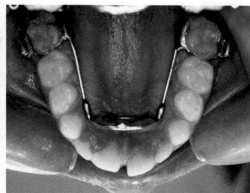

Figure 4.3 Fixed thumb guard to prevent digit sucking.

2000; Patel, 2008; Mistry *et al.*, 2010). These effects can be socially unacceptable and difficult to treat if left to establish in the permanent dentition.

There are a number of options to intercept the distortion effects of a digit habit, but children younger than 6 years of age are rarely able to cope with appliance treatment. Cognitive behavioural management with reward charts designed to reward 'good' rather than 'punish' bad behaviour are the interceptive measures of choice in the younger patient. If this has not been effective by 7 years of age, more definitive treatment is required and appliance therapy should be considered to ensure that arch distortion or displacement of the developing incisors does not occur. Simple measures such as nail paint, putting gloves on or finger/thumb splints can be used to deter the habit in patients who actively wish to give up. Appliance wear however can not only deter the habit, but can also be used to address other occlusal problems such as crossbites or overjet and overbite issues. For those who have a significant sagittal discrepancy, a functional appliance can be used to combine a deterrent with Class II correction. Unfortunately, any removable appliance can easily be removed at times when the urge to suck a digit is at its greatest (such as sitting in front of the TV or on long car journeys) and therefore is much less effective than an appliance that cannot be removed. The only true preventative appliance is the fixed thumb guard (Figure 4.3).

The fixed thumb guard ensures full compliance and is well tolerated. The wirework must be large enough to ensure the digit cannot be put into the mouth, thus forcing an immediate cessation of the habit, and it must be very well polished so that there is no trauma to the tongue. All habits are individual and there cannot be any general rule as to the period of wear; however, it is reasonable for these appliances to be left *in situ* for at least 6 months to ensure the habit is broken (Figure 4.4).

Fixed orthodontic expansion appliances, such as the Quadhelix, can also be used to incorporate arch expansion, but they are not as effective as a thumb guard as they do not physically stop the thumb from being put in the mouth (Figure 4.5). The design of these appliances should be modified so that the anterior wires act as a thumb guard.

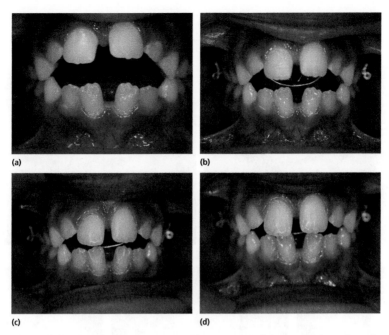

Figure 4.4 Clinical effects of the thumb guard. (a) Start. (b) At 3 months. (c) At 6 months. (d) At 9 months.

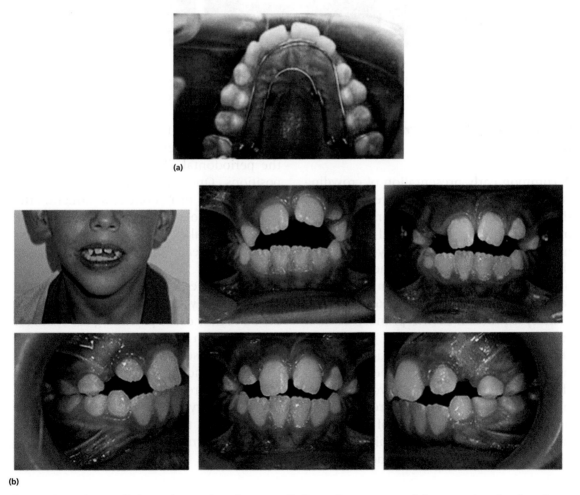

Figure 4.5 (a) The Quadhelix appliance. (b) Using a Quadhelix appliance to expand the upper dental arch and correct the lateral arch dimensions, as well as acting as a thumb guard.

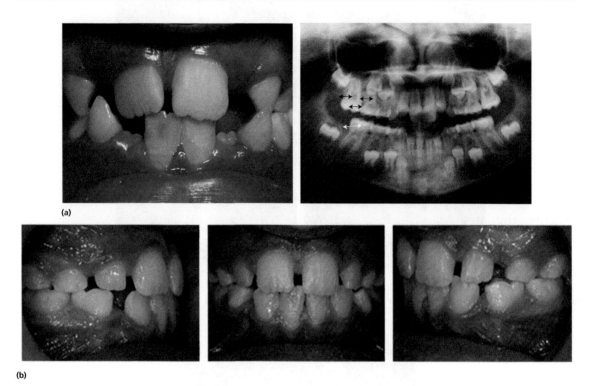

(a)

(b)

Figure 4.6 (a) Before extraction of the primary canines. (b) After extraction of the primary canines, space is created to allow the upper permanent lateral incisors to erupt, and the crowding is seen to shift distally in the arch.

Crowding of the permanent lateral incisors

A common early presentation of crowding is a lack of space for the development of the permanent lateral incisors. Delaying orthodontic treatment until all the permanent teeth have erupted may mean that these permanent teeth become rotated or displaced palatally, or even impacted, due to the lack of space (Figure 4.6).

Early extraction of the primary canines to create space to guide the eruption of these teeth has little evidence base; however, this approach can be justified if the consequences of the crowding for the patient are appreciated. If there is a shortage of space for the eruption of the permanent lateral incisors, it is certain that they will be displaced from their ideal position and orthodontic treatment will be necessary later. If they erupt rotated or displaced, the periodontal fibres form in these poor positions. Once the tooth position is corrected with orthodontic treatment, the fibres have to reorientate to stabilise the tooth. This takes a long time and often is incomplete, leading to the high probability of relapse of the tooth position or protracted retainer wear. More importantly, in today's society poor aesthetics is not tolerated and may cause psychological issues for the child with regard to self-esteem or lead to teasing at school.

Early extraction of primary canines to prevent centre-line shift is also indicated if one primary canine is lost early. For the best outcome the teeth should be removed before the permanent lateral incisors have erupted.

It must be understood that interceptive extractions will not eliminate crowding of the permanent dentition. In fact, they may make it worse as the lateral incisors will drift distally in the arch as they erupt. Early deciduous extraction is based on the premise that crowding of these teeth implies that there is a dento-alveolar disproportion and that extraction of a permanent unit in each quadrant is almost inevitable at a later date. This will normally be a premolar (usually the first premolar); however, exceptionally, it can be the permanent canine if this is ectopic, or indeed any other compromised tooth.

The great advantage of this interceptive approach is that anterior aesthetics is maintained throughout the establishment of the permanent dentition and the permanent teeth are guided into the dental arch form. This reduces the length of time of the later comprehensive orthodontic treatment in the established permanent dentition.

Other methods of inclusion of the lateral incisors will depend on the amount of crowding and the upper arch width. If there is minor crowding and an element of maxillary narrowness tending toward crossbite, upper arch expansion can be considered. The buccal segments should never be expanded into a buccal crossbite, but correcting posterior crossbites (with or without a displacement) to correct the arch shape and create space for the inclusion of all the adult dentition is valid (Figure 4.7).

Great care must be taken to ensure that the correct interdigitation of the buccal segments is maintained, and even if it is, long-term retention of this expansion will be required. However, in reality the whole argument about the importance of buccal segment interdigitation in retaining arch

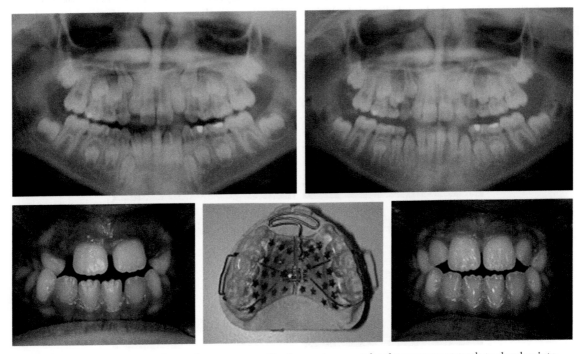

Figure 4.7 Early expansion can be used to create an effective environment for the permanent teeth to develop into.

expansion has to be challenged, as teeth are rarely together when at rest as there is a freeway space between the upper and lower dentition. The only time the teeth are in contact is during biting or tooth clenching and this amount of time cannot maintain the tooth position. It is much more likely that mild maxillary asymmetries are due to developmental moulding or tongue position.

If there is no buccal crossbite, expansion is not warranted and extraction of the primary canines or disking of them to create space for the lateral incisors to erupt is the treatment of choice. Choosing whether to undertake expansion of the arch or extraction of the teeth depends on a careful assessment of the patient. This will include radiographic examination with an orthopantogram (OPG), an assessment of the amount of crowding of the anterior teeth, the shape of the dental arch and the posterior occlusion, as well as consideration of the wishes of the child and their parents. The ability of the child to accept a

tooth extraction without being traumatised is also an important part of the treatment planning process. Good oral hygiene is an advantage and both the child and their parents must understand the long-term commitment to treatment and the possibility of further extractions and comprehensive orthodontic treatment at a later stage. This non-appliance approach is also particularly useful if no orthodontic treatment is contemplated or possible due to medical or physical factors, or even when compliance with oral hygiene is poor. The non-appliance guiding of the adult teeth into the line of the dental arch will usually give reasonable aesthetics without the need for complex orthodontic treatment.

Where there is little crowding but anterior spacing is leading to a lack of appropriate space for the developing secondary teeth, a short course of fixed appliance treatment to gather space in the upper labial segment can also have beneficial effects on the eruption of the secondary dentition (Figure 4.8).

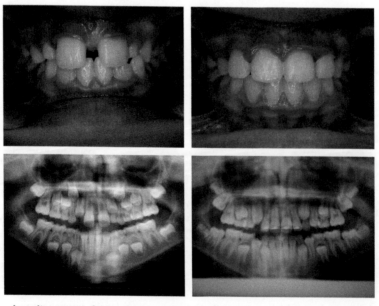

Figure 4.8 Using fixed appliances to close anterior incisor spacing early can be useful when guiding the developing dentition into the correct alignment.

Anterior crossbites

Anterior crossbites should be treated early to avoid periodontal damage, fenestration of the lower labial plate due to incisor displacement, tooth wear due to abnormal contact or mandibular displacement and the potential for temporomandibular joint (TMJ) dysfunction (Figures 4.9, 4.10 and 4.11). It is important to remember that the correction of anterior crossbites needs bite opening to avoid compensatory movement of the opposing teeth and therefore, bite planes may need to be used. As a removable appliance causes tipping movements of the teeth, it is preferable to begin correction of the crossbite early whilst the offending tooth is erupting as this takes advantage of the vertical movement of the tooth during treatment, which allows a better vector of movement of the tooth with the appliance during tooth eruption. If the tooth has fully erupted, further tipping will be required to correct its position. Once the tooth is in the correct position with a positive overbite, the bite blocks can be removed from the appliance as the crossbite will be self-retaining (Figures 4.12 and 4.13). It is important to ensure that adequate space is available for the labial movement of the tooth in crossbite. If there is no distal space for the teeth either side of the tooth in crossbite to be moved into, deciduous extractions will be necessary.

Occasionally, a crossbite can be corrected by extraction alone (Figure 4.14).

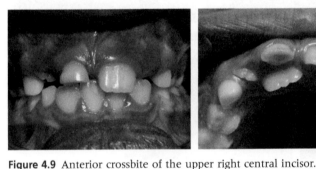
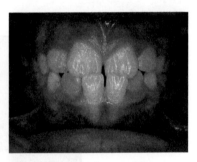

Figure 4.9 Anterior crossbite of the upper right central incisor.

Figure 4.10 Anterior crossbite causing forward displacement of the lower central incisors and leading to reduced labial bone coverage.

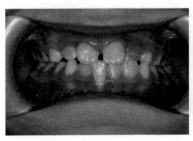
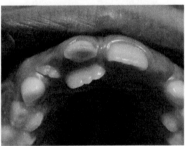
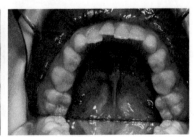

Figure 4.11 Case showing potential damage involving tooth wear and periodontal involvement.

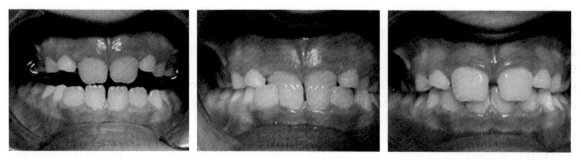

Figure 4.12 When correcting an anterior crossbite, posterior coverage is needed to open the bite beyond the depth of the crossbite.

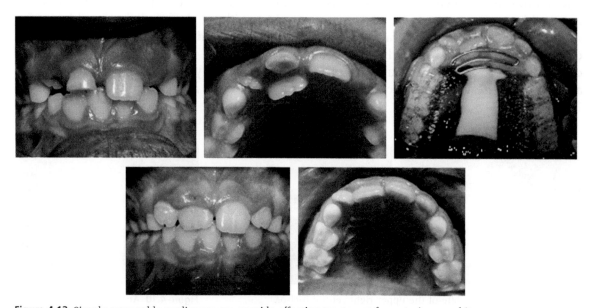

Figure 4.13 Simple removable appliances can provide effective treatment for anterior crossbites.

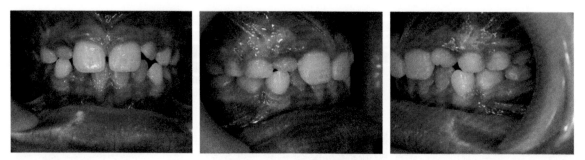

Figure 4.14 Extraction of the lower canines eliminates the crossbite.

Posterior crossbites and guidance of the secondary dentition

Expansion of the posterior teeth is a contentious subject. There is little evidence to confirm that early expansion in the absence of a crossbite will create enough space for the permanent teeth to develop into and improve the arch form, or that a crossbite is damaging to dental or TMJ health. However, if a number of features are present, such as a crossbite, displacement and asymmetrical dental arch form, expansion has the potential to guide the developing secondary dentition and, in cases with mild crowding, of eliminating the need for extractions by producing a symmetrical dental arch.

Before embarking on expansion, careful assessment of an OPG is required. Although an accurate space analysis cannot be done from a tomograph, a rough space assessment can be done by measuring the space between the distal edge of the lateral incisor and first permanent molar (including an assessment of any anterior spacing that can be used to accommodate the teeth) and comparing this with the combined crown widths of the canine and both premolars. The difference will give a good idea of whether the crowding is mild, moderate or severe. Careful assessment of the OPG will also rule out the presence of hypodontia or supernumerary teeth, which may significantly influence early deciduous arch guidance.

Posterior expansion can be done with a removable or fixed appliance (Figures 4.15 and 4.16), but care must be taken to ensure the bite is opened with posterior bite blocks on removable appliances, or Glass Ionomer cement placed on the teeth when using a Quadhelix appliance to avoid compensatory expansion of the lower arch due to the cuspal interlock. Appliances should be worn full-time during the active phase and for at least 6 months afterwards to allow the arch dimension to stabilise. It is usually preferable to use a fixed appliance rather than a removable one as compliance is guaranteed if the appliance cannot be removed by the patient. This treatment works well for arches where the crossbite is due to dental or dento-alveolar malposition. When the crossbite is skeletal in origin, expansion of a narrow maxilla will not be stable.

A number of practitioners take the view that arch expansion should be undertaken in most circumstances to accommodate all the permanent teeth. They claim that this approach will give a broad arch that is both aesthetic and functional. However, there is no respected evidence to confirm this and no long-term studies that demonstrate that arch expansion will be stable if there is intrinsic dento-alveolar disproportion. When expansion is done in these circumstances, long-term or even life-long retention is required. For an adult who is looking for a specific aesthetic solution, this may not be unreasonable, but for a child, expansion of the maxillary arch (when there is no crossbite) often requires concomitant expansion of the mandibular arch. Without clear soft tissue factors indicating that this is advisable, long periods of retainer wear will be required, which is an unrealistic expectation for a child.

There is a need for a period of retainer wear after most orthodontic tooth movements. The important question is how long is it reasonable to expect a child to wear a retainer. Commitment to retainer wear must be part of informed consent, but expanding the dental arches in the knowledge that they will be unstable or expecting

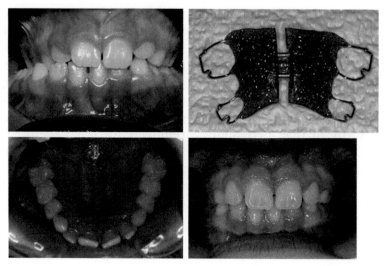

Figure 4.15 Upper arch expansion with a removable appliance to eliminate a unilateral crossbite.

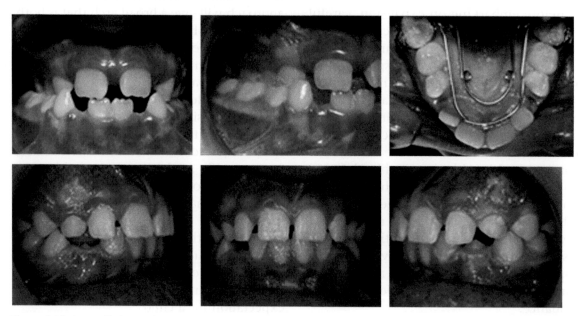

Figure 4.16 A Quadhelix appliance can eliminate the need for patient compliance as it is not removable from the mouth.

that the soft tissues or skeletal bases will expand with the dental movements is bad practice. It is of course impossible on an individual basis to assess this, but the greater the expansion the more likely it is that it will relapse. As in all orthodontic treatment planning, there are guidelines but very little absolute evidence on which to base specific practice. A full discussion with the patient, a cautious approach and excellent mechanics is the most likely recipe for success.

Serial extraction: a modern approach

Serial extraction was introduced in the 1940s to guide the developing dentition at a time when orthodontic appliances did not easily allow precise tooth movement. Its practice fell out of favour with the introduction of sophisticated fixed appliance systems in the 1970s as it was thought that these simplified the approach to orthodontic treatment. More recently, due to the demand for higher aesthetic standards during the developing dentition phase, an appreciation has developed for the advantages of interceptive tooth guidance and as a result there has been a decline in fixed appliance treatment.

The modern approach starts with the removal of the primary canines in cases where there is anterior crowding to allow the permanent incisors to align as the lateral incisors are erupting (Figure 4.17a). This is usually undertaken at 7–8 years of age. This is followed by a period of occlusal monitoring (Figure 4.17b). As the first premolars erupt at around 10 years of age, the position of the permanent canines is assessed and if crowding is present, the first premolars are removed to allow the eruption of the canines and second premolars into the line of the dental arch (Figure 4.17c). When serial extraction was first described, the first deciduous molars were also extracted, but there is no evidence that they delay the eruption of the first premolars. It is felt that this is an unnecessary stage in the process. During occlusal management with interceptive extractions, the occlusion should be reassessed every 9–12 months until the permanent dentition has erupted (Figure 4.17d). If the permanent tooth position is not ideal, fixed appliances can be placed to improve the tooth position. If the tooth position is acceptable or the oral hygiene is poor, this interceptive approach will hopefully lead to the reasonable alignment of the teeth without the need for fixed appliance therapy.

The premise behind this approach is to use the natural eruptive potential of the teeth to improve tooth position rather than allowing teeth to move ectopically before orthodontic treatment. This approach can significantly shorten the active treatment time. In cases where there is a skeletal element to the malocclusion, serial extraction can be combined with sagittal correction with headgear or functional appliances. When the skeletal discrepancy cannot be managed with functional appliances, masking of the overjet can be done by extraction of the first premolars in the maxilla and allowing proclination of the lower labial segment to manage any crowding in the lower arch. This approach will have implications for retention and must be discussed with the patient.

Modern occlusal guidance is geared towards encouraging the permanent dentition to erupt into the line of the dental arch with selective extractions (Figure 4.18). If a tooth is very ectopic (particularly a canine), it may be more expedient to remove this tooth, and thereby avoid the need to commit the patient to many months of complex orthodontics to pull the tooth into the line of the arch. With modern restorative materials and adhesive dentistry, very good camouflage and crown modification can be achieved.

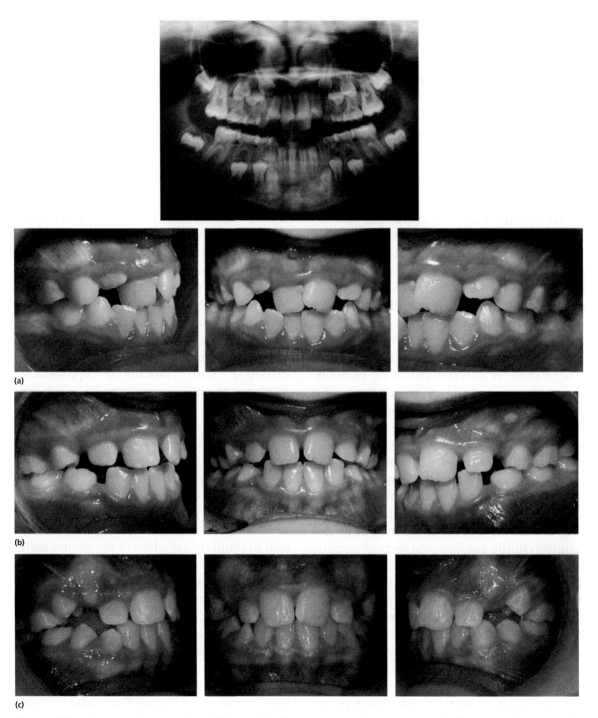

Figure 4.17 Serial extraction. (a) Start. (b) 6 months after primary canine extraction. (c) First premolars erupted and ready for extraction. (d) Second premolars erupting, ready for alignment if required.

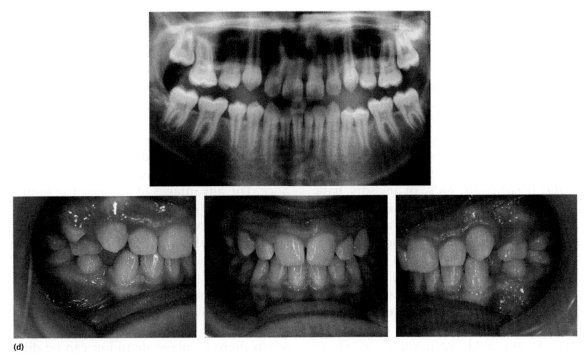

(d)

Figure 4.17 (*Continued*)

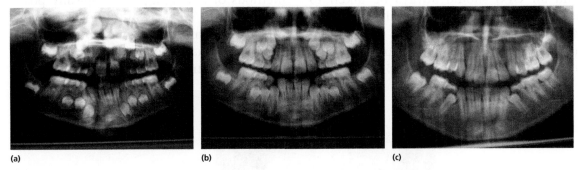

(a)   (b)   (c)

Figure 4.18 Series of OPG radiographs showing the management of severe crowding with interceptive extractions alone, thus avoiding the need for orthodontic treatment. (a) 2009; (b) 2011; (c) 2014.

The unerupted central incisor

If the eruption of one central incisor is more than 6 months delayed with respect to the other or the lateral incisor has erupted, it is important to take radiographs to assess its position (Mason *et al.*, 2000). The most common cause of delayed eruption is the presence of a supernumerary tooth (Figure 4.19) (DiBiase, 1968–1969). After removal of the obstruction, 68% of incisors have been shown to erupt spontaneously (if there is sufficient space in the arch) within 12 months (Witsenberg and Boering, 1981). It is prudent however, to bond a gold chain to the unerupted tooth at the time of the surgical removal of the supernumerary(s) to ensure a second procedure is avoided if there is no spontaneous eruption; if there is, the gold chain simply needs to be removed. Careful clinical assessment is required with palpation buccally and palatally. Radiographic examination should include either vertical or horizontal parallax depending on the radiographs taken, and an OPG should always be taken to assess all the developing dentition (Figure 4.20). Cone-beam computed tomography (CBCT) is also an invaluable tool in assessing tooth position (see Figure 3.4).

If a tooth is impeded in its eruption, this may be due to an obstruction or dilaceration of the root. If either is the case, the tooth is unlikely to erupt on its own, but could be brought into place with orthodontic traction even if severely ectopic (Figures 4.21 and 4.22).

This treatment however can be very protracted and careful discussion with the patient is needed to ensure their compliance. The advantages of bringing the tooth into the line of the arch is that alveolar bone is preserved and will be brought into the area as the tooth moves. With this approach, the resulting contour of the gingival margin is likely to be better with respect to the other incisors than that achieved with a bridge or implant. Bringing an unerupted tooth down at a young age when there is mixed dentition can be difficult and protracted, and the root of the dilacerated tooth can become compromised. Each case must be assessed on its own merits and skeletal pattern and smile line must be taken into account. Other methods of managing an ectopically positioned tooth, such as autotransplantation of crowded premolars or the unerupted tooth itself, have been tried with varying results. With transplantation, the problems

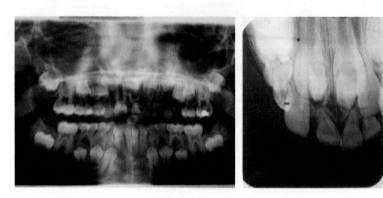

Figure 4.19 Tuberculate supernumeraries preventing the eruption of the central incisors.

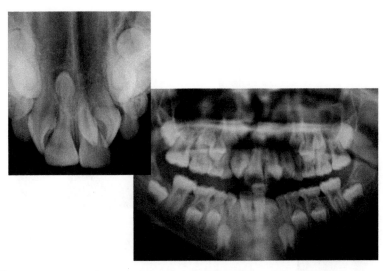

Figure 4.20 Mesiodens supernumeraries preventing the eruption of the central incisors.

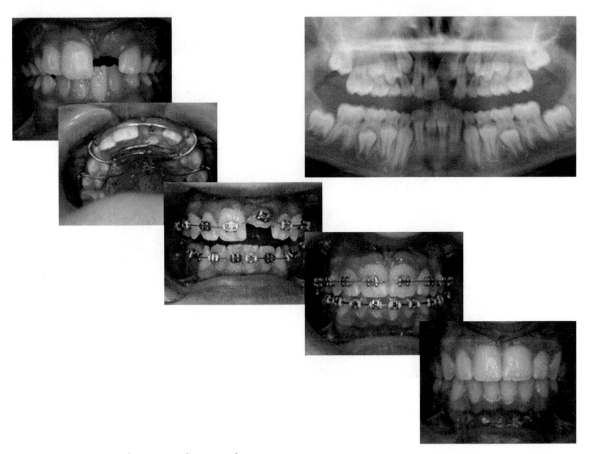

Figure 4.21 Managing the impacted incisor: the treatment sequence.

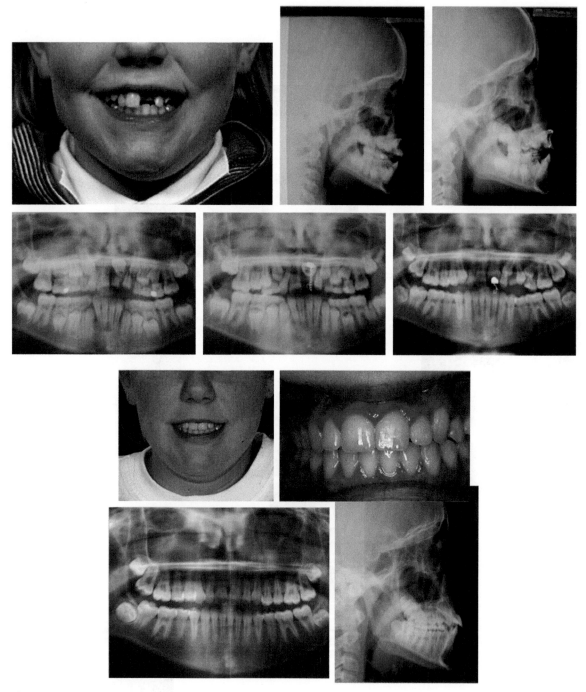

Figure 4.22 Severely ectopic teeth can be effectively treated with complex orthodontic treatment. Bringing the teeth into the line of the dental arch preserves alveolar bone.

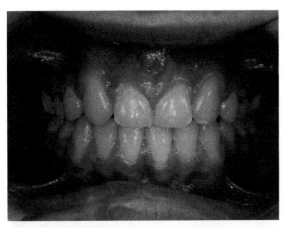

Figure 4.23 Lateral incisor moved into central incisor position and restored showing poor emergence profile.

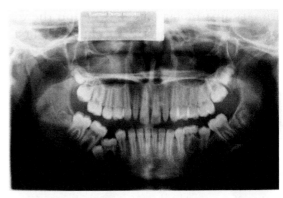

Figure 4.24 Submerging lower right second deciduous molar and impacted second premolar.

of devitalisation, gingival margin contour and ankylosis must be considered.

Attempting to move the lateral incisor into the central incisor space is also possible and useful if there has been early space loss or there is an increased overjet that requires incisor retraction. The disadvantage of this approach, however, is that the emerging profile of the lateral incisor is usually narrow at the gingival margin, which often leads to poor aesthetics and difficulty with cleaning (Czochrowska *et al.*, 2003) (Figure 4.23). The level of the smile line, alveolar bone level and patient preference will significantly influence the space closure method of choice.

Nowadays the success of single tooth implants often makes this the option of choice; however, an implant cannot be placed until growth has stopped, and the child will have either to wear a retainer to hold the space open or have an acid-etched retained bridge (AERB) placed. The AERB is of course a more stable option as it is not removable from the mouth, but it must be well looked after and demands high oral hygiene standards from the child.

Submerging deciduous second molars

The evidence for the management of these teeth is limited; however, guidance is that if there is a successor, it will usually exfoliate (Ericson and Kurol, 1988a; Power and Short, 1993; Baccetti *et al.*, 2008).

In treatment planning, consideration needs to be given to the presence or absence of crowding, the severity of the submergence and the periodontal condition. An OPG radiograph should always be taken to assess for the presence of a successional tooth under the submerging tooth and whether it is in an ectopic position (Figure 4.24). Extraction of the second deciduous molar can lead to space loss (particularly in a crowded arch) and possible impaction of the developing second premolar if present. This could lead to a food trap and eventual periodontal damage; therefore, early detection and treatment planning are important (Figure 4.25). Where space loss is expected, a space maintainer can be considered. Previously, band and loop styles have been advocated, but these are difficult to make and often do not control the space as the primary first molar may be lost and therefore, there is no mesial stop and the first permanent molar tilts forward (Figure 4.26). In these cases a lower lingual arch

should be placed (Figure 4.27) or a decision made that the crowding is sufficient to allow the space to be lost with the plan to extract one premolar in the future.

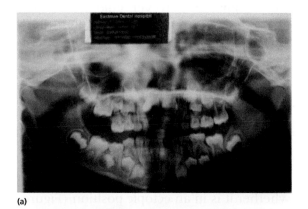

Figure 4.25 Submerging lower left second deciduous molar causing a food trap.

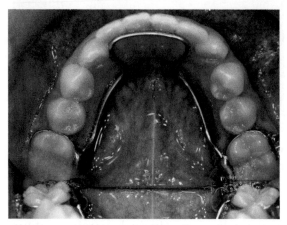

Figure 4.27 A lingual arch is effective at stabilising the molar position and arch length after loss of a primary second molar.

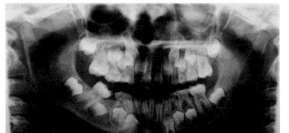

(a)

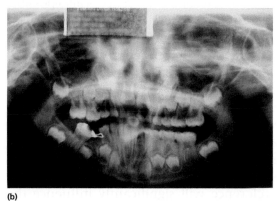

(b)

(c)

Figure 4.26 A band and loop is rarely successful in preventing the medial tipping of the first molar after loss of primary molars. (a) Before extraction of the primary second molar. (b) Band and loop in place, but not controlling mesial movement of the adult molar. (c) Loss of space leading to impaction of the developing premolars.

Fusion, gemination and morphology issues

'Large teeth' of any aetiology are best managed early if possible to ensure that there is as little disruption to the rest of the developing dentition as possible (Figure 4.28). The normal size of the upper incisors is 9 mm and by using the 'golden proportion' of 1:0.64; this means that a lateral incisor is usually 6.5 mm. The size of the root and pulp chamber is critical in deciding if the abnormally sized tooth can be reduced aesthetically. Fused or geminated teeth rarely do well if they are sectioned as the periodontal tissues are compromised and ankylosis is common. Careful planning with consideration of the malocclusion as a whole must be undertaken, and if a tooth is removed, great care must be taken to avoid displacement of the dental centre line, as this does not improve aesthetics and is difficult to correct later. If space is not corrected, the development of the lateral incisors will be affected. These incisors are often impacted, displaced or rotated, which can lead to significant difficulties later on (Figure 4.29). If the size of the tooth allows, the crown should be reduced, but this approach very much depends on the root and pulp chamber widths as well as the crown. The amount of enamel to be reduced cannot be so large that it necessitates tooth reduction into the dentine as this will be sensitive. If tooth reduction is not possible, consideration should be given to removing one of the oversized incisors and using a sectional fixed appliance to move the remaining incisor into a position where it can be built up to mimic the size of two normal incisors (Figure 4.30). The single tooth can then be aesthetically contoured to make it look like two crowns and thus preserve aesthetics and tooth tissue proportions. Once the lateral incisors have erupted, aesthetics is usually reasonable and later orthodontic treatment can be undertaken (including the removal of the last central incisor) to localise space appropriately for a permanent restoration of the upper labial segment with either a bridge or implant. This option helps to preserve alveolar bone for implant provision later on, but will require consultation with a restorative specialist to plan the final restorations.

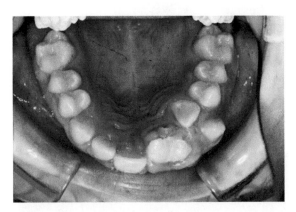

Figure 4.28 A geminated central incisor.

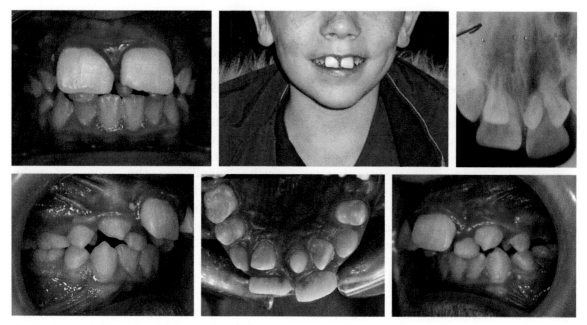

Figure 4.29 Large upper central incisors (megadont teeth) cause occlusal issues and crowding due to their size, and benefit from early management.

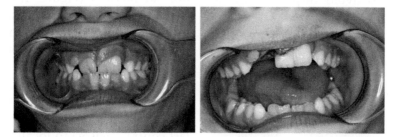

Figure 4.30 Orthodontic tooth movement and restorative management of one megadont tooth to allow space for normal occlusal development of the remaining incisors.

Upper labial fraenum

A large upper labial fraenum can cause a median diastema and can become traumatised with tooth brushing or eating (Figure 4.31). As part of a long-term orthodontic plan, a prominent labial fraenum is often removed if large or demonstrated to have fibre attachments into the incisive foramen. There is little agreement as to whether removal is better before or after orthodontic treatment. On one hand it is difficult to

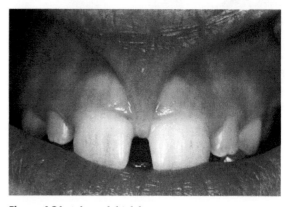

Figure 4.31 A large labial fraenum.

remove all the tissue if the upper incisors are in contact with one another, but if the fraenum is removed early with the incisors apart, it is suggested that scar tissue makes diastema closure and retention difficult. In most cases, the decision is left to the individual clinician, the demands of the malocclusion or the wishes of the patient/parents.

Lip traps

Lip traps (Figures 4.32 and 4.33) can cause displacement of the teeth and are often signs of an underlying skeletal discrepancy. They can be treated early to avoid unwanted tooth movement, but care must be taken to ensure that unwanted effects, such as converting a Class II/1 incisor relationship into a Class II/2 relationship due to the underlying skeletal discrepancy. Early treatment may be necessary to ensure that the risk of trauma to the proclined teeth is avoided, but will necessitate a long-term orthodontic commitment. Patients may wish for early intervention on aesthetic grounds and should be fully informed of the prognosis with varying severity of skeletal pattern.

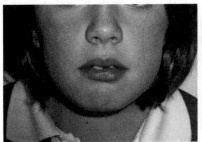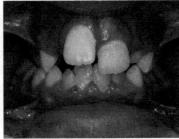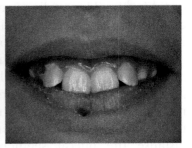

Figure 4.32 Lip trap causing proclination of incisors.

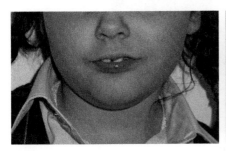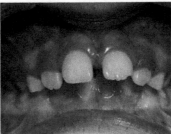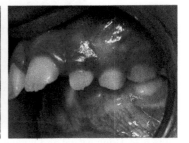

Figure 4.33 Lip trap causing proclination of the upper central incisors and retroclination of the lower incisors.

Leeway space and the use of intraoral anchorage arches

The leeway space is the size differential between the primary posterior teeth (canine, first and second molars) and the permanent successors. The sum of the primary tooth widths is normally greater than that of their permanent successors. When the primary teeth exfoliate, there is usually an excess of space (about 2.5 mm on either side in the lower arch and 1.5 mm on either side in the upper arch). If nothing is done to preserve this space, the permanent first molars will drift forward to close it. In Class I cases, this leads to the establishment of the stable Class I molar relationship. If mild crowding is evident in the dental arch, it is possible to utilise this space difference to avoid extractions (Brennan and Gianelly, 2000). By placing a lingual or palatal arch before the exfoliation of the primary second molar, the first permanent molar is limited in its natural mesial migration and fixed appliances can be used to distalise the buccal segment teeth and canines when they erupt (Ngan *et al.*, 2000; Zablocki *et al.*, 2008) (Figure 4.34). This allows the elimination of mild anterior incisor crowding without the use of extractions or interdental stripping. In the lower arch, a lingual arch fixes the arch length between the molars and lower incisors, and the arch length is then secure. In the upper arch, the overbite may not allow for the placement of a wire behind the upper incisors and a palatal arch with a nance button may have to be used. Control of the arch length in this situation is less effective but still useful.

If crowding is assessed as moderate on the OPG (with a skeletal Class I or II pattern), then preserving the leeway space may not be in the patient's best interest, and planning for the extraction of premolar units may be the best option so that tooth movement can be achieved with plenty of anchorage. If the skeletal pattern is Class II and anchorage is at a premium, holding the molars back may prove useful for future orthodontics.

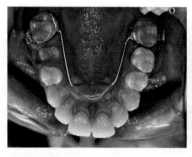 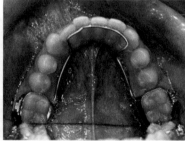

Figure 4.34 Using palatal and lingual arches to preserve the leeway space.

Sagittal problems: Class II

A great deal of research has been undertaken into the effects of sagittal correction using either functional or fixed appliances. The majority of the evidence shows that with this treatment there is often minimal skeletal change combined with a much larger dental and alveolar change. Studies have shown that the rate of treatment change may be quicker during the pubertal growth spurt, but none has been able to answer the questions whether this change is more stable in the long term and whether or not the skeletal growth would in any event have achieved the same position (even if not the dental relationship) at the end of the growth period (Tulloch *et al.*, 1998; O'Brien *et al.*, 2009). This debate is well covered elsewhere and is open to much controversy, but it is important for a clinician to look at more than the growth evidence when choosing the ideal time for introducing sagittal treatment.

There is evidence that more than 40% of children with large overjets (Figure 4.35) of more than 8mm will traumatise their incisors (Figure 4.36) and, although the peak incidence of trauma to the incisors is in toddlers (2–4 years of age), there is good evidence that there is a second peak at 7–9 years of age when the permanent succes-

sors are present. This trauma can lead to permanent injury to the incisors. This fact, combined with an improvement in dental aesthetics if the upper incisors are within lip control, should be the driving force for early treatment.

Many objections to early treatment have been made, such as the difficulties young patients have with complying with treatment and the length of the process. In reality, the younger patient does very well with early treatment. At 8–9 years of age, compliance with appliances is often excellent as the challenges of adolescence have yet to become apparent. Bringing the incisors out of danger will reduce the likelihood of injury and may improve social contact

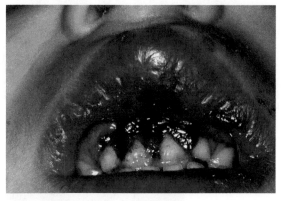

Figure 4.36 Result of a fall, fracture and luxation of the anterior teeth.

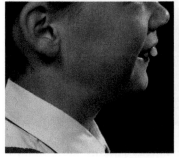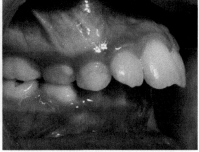

Figure 4.35 Proclination of the upper incisors increases the risk of trauma.

and reduce teasing, even if it does not correct the overall malocclusion. Psychologically, children have been shown to derive significant benefits from early treatment in terms of increased self-concept scores and reduced negative social experiences with improved self-esteem and improved facial profile (Vig and Vig, 1986) (Figure 4.37). This early treatment can be combined with extractions if there is dento-alveolar disproportion, and a second phase of treatment with fixed appliance alignment of the teeth once the

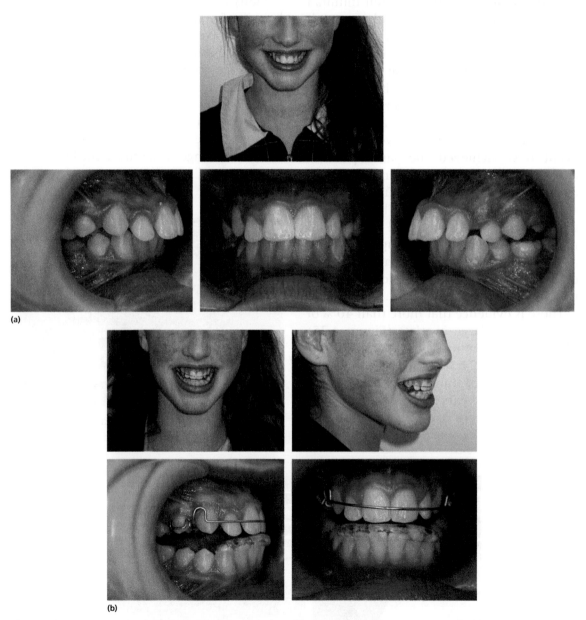

Figure 4.37 A treatment sequences for the management of an increased overjet. (a) Start. (b) With the appliance in place. (c) Post treatment with the overjet reduced.

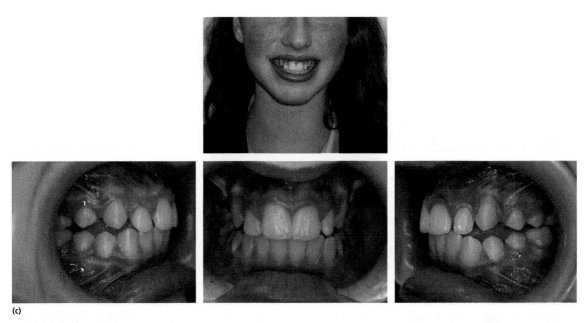

(c)

Figure 4.37 (*Continued*)

permanent dentition has established can be used to manage long-term occlusal needs (Fränkel, 1966). However, this early treatment should not replace comprehensive orthodontic treatment to correct a malocclusion. It may be that the skeletal discrepancy is too great or does not respond to the functional appliance forces. Rotations and severe crowding cannot be resolved at this young age, but a young patient can gain many benefits from the elimination of a lip trap and the retroclination of prominent incisors. The very act of placing a functional appliance in the mouth of someone with a large overjet reduces it and produces better facial balance. This alone is of great benefit to some patients and reinforces compliance. There are of course many compromises in this style of treatment and it is not for all. If the young patient feels overwhelmed by wearing a functional appliance or there is not the parental support necessary for this style of treatment, there is little chance of success. If the appliance is not well made, it will be difficult or painful to wear and probably not tolerated. If instructions are not clear or follow-up not supportive, it will be difficult to inspire confidence in the patient or parents.

The tooth movements with this early treatment follow the same pattern as with all functional appliance therapy. If there is the potential for mandibular growth, the mandible will grow. If not, there will be dental movement to camouflage the skeletal discrepancy. This of course may not be stable in the long term, but this initial treatment is often hugely advantageous for aesthetics and greatly appreciated by the patient. No guarantees can be given at the start of treatment, but careful management of the appliance, patient and parents can often lead to a very positive improvement. If a lip trap is eliminated in cases with a mild skeletal discrepancy by retroclination of the upper incisors and mild proclination of the lower incisors, this may remain stable after the initial treatment with the soft tissues

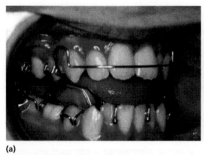 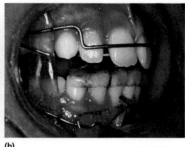 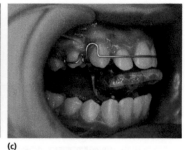

(a)   (b)   (c)

Figure 4.38 Functional appliances come in many designs but generally effect the same outcome. (a) Clark Twin Block; (b) functional regulator II; and (c) median opening activator.

controlling the tooth position. If there is any skeletal change, this can only benefit the patient, but should not be guaranteed during the initial treatment discussion.

There is no conclusive evidence to confirm that early treatment is effective as a reduction in the overjet could be due to acceleration of mandibular growth or just posture. It is also not possible to predict how much of the reduction will still be present at 14–15 years of age or, on an individual basis, to distinguish whether any treatment changes are due to natural growth or the effects of the appliance.

While this treatment is not for all, it is often successful and improves aesthetics, reduces the risk of incisor trauma and improves self-esteem without being too arduous for the patient. It is also reversible and non-injurious, and easy for the patient to stop treatment at any time should they wish. For these reasons, it is a treatment option that should be offered to all patients with Class II/1 malocclusions where there is patient or parent concern.

Once the initial objectives of treatment have been achieved (and if the appliance is worn as instructed there will *always* be a reduction in the overjet), the difficulty is maintaining any change. With a good anterior oral seal, the overjet reduction may be

self-retaining, but if (as is often the case in young children) there is a lip apart posture at rest, the overjet will return if there is poor compliance with retention. This is usually by managed by wearing the appliance for nights only. When deciding on the type of appliance, it is very important to consider that there may be deciduous teeth exfoliating during the active treatment phase, the depth of the overbite, any crowding present and the needs of the patient. There are many types of appliance such as activators, Fränkel appliances, hybrid appliances and those that produce specific changes such as intrusive activators (Figure 4.38). Careful case assessment is essential before choosing the appliance for each individual.

Functional appliances use the muscles of mastication to change the relationship between the maxillary and mandibular dentition. They harness the force of the stretched masticatory muscles and transfer this to the teeth and supporting structures. Functional appliances can be fixed or removable, but at very young ages fixed appliances are inappropriate as deciduous teeth may be exfoliating and these appliances are also difficult for young patients to tolerate. All of the currently used appliances are assemblies of components. The details of these components vary qualitatively and quantitatively, as does the configuration of the connecting elements and hence the overall appearance of the appliance (Vig and Vig, 1986).

The ideal appliance for very young patients is the functional regulator (FRII) developed by Fränkel (1966) (Figure 4.39). It is ideal for the developing dentition as there are no physical attachments to the teeth. The FRII uses the linguo-facial muscle balance with shields deflecting the soft tissues and bite planes to guide the eruption of the teeth, and the forward posture of the mandible to change the incisor position. The sagittal jaw relationship changes are achieved by a combination of effects such as tipping of incisors, inhibition of mesial migration of maxillary teeth, mesial movement of mandibular teeth, inhibition of maxillary alveolar height increase and extrusion of mandibular molars, inhibition of forward growth of the maxilla, increased growth of the mandible, as well as changes in condylar growth direction and amount. If an appliance is worn well, the overjet will reduce (either by skeletal or dento-alveolar movement) and the stability is dependent on the severity of the initial skeletal deformity, its response to treatment and the degree to which the incisors are controlled by the soft tissues. Profile improvement only occurs if there has been skeletal change. Patients who achieve good outcomes with this style of treatment usually have mild skeletal discrepancies and no abnormal soft tissue factors, and they must be able to comply with treatment. If a patient has a severe skeletal discrepancy or does not manage to wear the appliance full-time, they rarely do well.

A detailed assessment, clear realistic objectives and rigorous management can improve the odds of a successful outcome.

An overall impression of facial form and head posture as well as the facial pattern of the child and both parents must be considered. Soft tissue influences (lip tone, lip competence, lip and mentalis muscle activity) and the height of the lip line are also important.

Before treatment it must be decided how much change is required and will meet the patient's wishes, as well as consideration of their ability to cooperate. It is also important for the clinician to be willing to reassess and adjust the appliance during treatment as changes occur.

Practical aspects
Functional bite registration
The aim of treatment is to achieve an edge-to-edge incisor position if possible, but if the overjet is severe or the patient is emotionally too young, it may be better to achieve this in two stages with the patient posturing as far as they can and then asking the patient to relax and reduce the amount of posture by a millimetre or so for comfort. The amount of opening depends on the overbite and face height. The deeper the bite, the greater the opening should be to allow for buccal segment eruption. It should be remembered that the functional appliance in this context is being used as an interceptive appliance, not a definitive appliance, and the objectives must be limited accordingly to ensure that a young patient can wear the appliance with some comfort. Wax impressions should include the full sulcus depth and the bite registration to allow for specific positioning (Figure 4.40).

First fit
It is important to ensure that the appliance is well made and there are no rough edges. The child and their parents should be given written instructions specific to

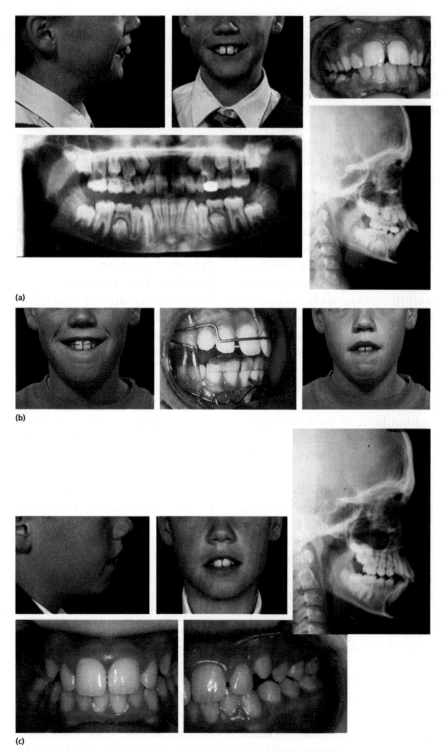

Figure 4.39 A treatment sequence for the management of an increased overjet. (a) Start. (b) A usual regimen is for an active phase of 9–12 months, followed by a passive phase of night-time wear only. Once in, the appliance is unobtrusive and there is an instant 'Class II' correction, which many children find very helpful. (c) The end result can be very rewarding for the patient, their parents and the practitioner.

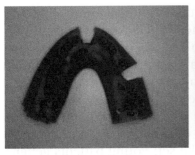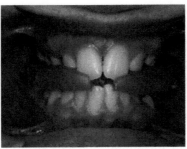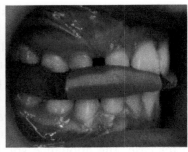

Figure 4.40 Using dental wax to provide a postured position for a functional appliance.

their appliance and needs, and for it to be demonstrated that the patient can place the appliance by themselves. It is important to explain about the effects on speech and excessive initial salivation. It is also essential that the child understands that wearing the appliance is their responsibility. Wear time should be set at an achievable level; this could be part-time for the first few days to allow a young child to get used to the appliance before encouraging full-time wear. Care of the appliance should be discussed, as well as what to do if breakages occur or it is lost.

Day-to-day management

Functional appliances should be removed for meals, sport and cleaning, and when not in the mouth *must* be placed in the storage box.

About 1–2 mm of overjet reduction per month can be expected and, if the appliance was not fully advanced at the start of treatment, it must be reactivated. The aim should be that by the end of treatment, the closest possible edge-to-edge incisor relationship should be achieved. The child should be aware that if compliance is poor, the clinician will not be fooled.

The timing of the end of treatment will be dictated by the reduction in overjet, compliance of the child and the wishes of

the family. This style of treatment does not aim to definitively treat the malocclusion, so it is important not to overreach the objectives initially set. Once the overjet is reduced, the amount of time spent wearing the appliance should be reduced to nights-only wear. Functional treatment should not last more than 6–9 months.

Dealing with poor compliance

It is important to remember that treatment is for the patient, not the orthodontist or parents. It is important to give 'honourable' ways out if a young child cannot cope with the appliance. As more treatment is likely to be needed later, it is important to build respect. The clinician should be prepared to stop treatment for an agreed period if it is getting too much, but the downside of non-compliance should be clearly stated.

One strategy to manage the poor complier who will not admit they are not wearing the appliance, and particularly when the parents insist that the child is wearing the appliance, is the 3 month–6 month rule. The clinician should tell the parents that (for fear of causing some dental damage) the appliance should be stopped as it is unheard of for an appliance that is worn regularly not to move the teeth and there is now concern that the child's bone may be abnormal. This elicits one of two responses. If the child and parents are unwilling to comply, they will accept this decision. If they do wish to continue treatment, the child (and often the parents) will admit that they may be able to wear the appliance for a little longer each day and ask to have the appliance returned. In the latter case, the appliance should be given back with a comment that if there is no movement by 6 months, treatment will stop. This has to be adhered to. Behavioural management is essential in all appliance therapy and particularly in treatments that involve appliances that can be removed from the mouth. If it is necessary to stop treatment after 6 months, there will be another opportunity to treat the child when older either with another functional appliance or extractions. For this reason, early cessation of treatment is often important if the child is struggling.

Involving the parents

It is important to involve the parents but also to ensure they understand they are not the ones being treated. It is often a good idea for the parents of young patients to be in the surgery for support and to ensure that any instructions are fully understood. However, parents should not be used by the orthodontist to punish their child for non-compliance. The orthodontist should be the one to manage the child's compliance with treatment; the parents will have more than enough other battles to overcome with their child.

The struggling child

Goals should be set; young patients generally wish to please. If they struggle initially to wear an appliance, encouragement and support is appropriate. Eventually however, if it is claimed that an appliance is being worn but there is no improvement, the clinician must take a firmer approach. This situation is particularly difficult if both the parents and child are adamant that the appliance is being worn, but there are no clinical signs of improvement.

It must be remembered that if a functional appliance is worn, the overjet will always reduce. Even when there is no skeletal or mandibular posture change, there will (by the action of the Class II effect) be changes in the inclination of the incisors. The upper incisors will retrocline and the lower incisors procline. Thus, the only reason for no change in overjet during treatment is inadequate wear of the appliance. These changes occur in non-growing individuals just as they do in children.

Sagittal problems: Class III
(Figure 4.41)

It is important with Class III patients to monitor the growth of the maxilla and mandible carefully. Early protraction headgear or chincup therapy can be useful, although if the skeletal discrepancy is large it may be difficult to achieve good aesthetics. Dento-alveolar camouflage of a Class III incisor relationship will depend on the severity of the malocclusion of the skeletal bases, but may be worth undertaking for aesthetic reasons even if complete correction cannot be achieved. Interceptive alignment of a crowded upper arch in a severe skeletal Class III patient is often important during adolescence for social acceptance, even if the ultimate treatment plan is orthognathic surgery (Bailey *et al.*, 1999).

It is highly unlikely that skeletal modification is stable with early treatment. Protraction of the maxilla with facemasks or restraint of the mandible with a chincup will have effects during the treatment phase, but they will not be long lasting. Growth of the skeletal bases is under genetic control and cannot be significantly changed. Dento-alveolar movement will mask a mild skeletal discrepancy, but this can be achieved just as well with fixed appliances and Class III traction elastics (Figure 4.42).

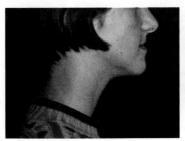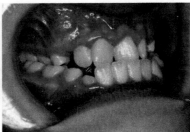

Figure 4.41 Class III malocclusion.

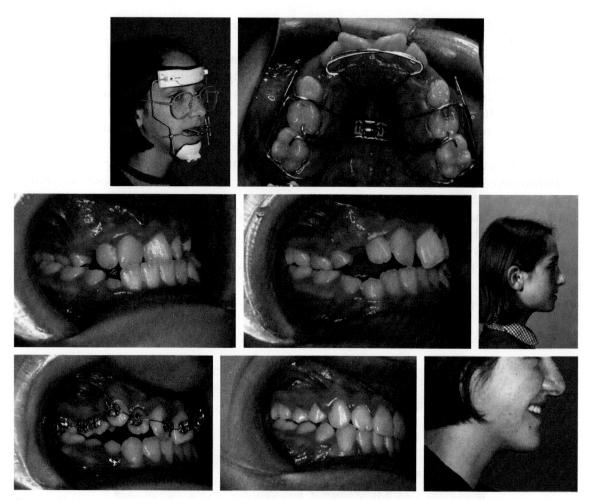

Figure 4.42 The treatment of Class III malocclusion with protraction headgear and fixed appliances.

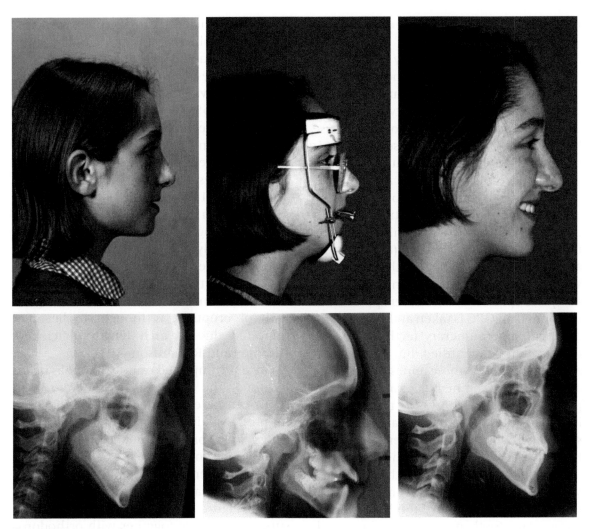

Figure 4.42 (*Continued*)

Ectopic and impacted teeth

Any tooth can be ectopically placed. The commonest ectopic tooth in the developing child is the upper canine. Guidance with early extraction of the primary canines is a common management protocol. Its use however is based on weak scientific evidence, and careful assessment of the position of the canine vertically and towards the mid-line is important to ensure the effectiveness of this intervention. All children should be assessed clinically as the upper central incisors erupt (at about the age of 7 years) to ensure that the adult incisors are in the correct position and there is adequate space for them to erupt without rotation. If an OPG is taken at this stage, not only can supernumerary teeth and odontomes often be identified, but the position and angulation of the canines also can be assessed. If the canine bulge cannot be palpated and an OPG shows the teeth are not in a good position, an upper standard occlusal radiograph should be taken to identify the labio-palatal position of the tooth.

An impacted tooth is a tooth that is prevented from erupting into its normal functional position by bone, tooth or fibrous tissue. Any tooth may become impacted: the third molars, canines, second premolars and incisors (Ericson and Kurol, 1988b). Impacted third molars are common (approx. 25%), but these teeth are not within the scope of this book. The incidence of impaction of second premolars is also high (Collett, 2000), whilst the incidence of impaction of the rest of the dentition is low.

The canine tooth is considered to be the 'cornerstone' tooth of the arch and is needed for protection of the occlusion via canine guidance. It is seldom extracted unless the prognosis for bringing it into the line of the arch is very poor. If the canine becomes impacted, treatment often involves a multidisciplinary approach and a long time. The quoted incidence of impacted canines varies from 0.9% to 3.3%. It is more than twice as common in females as in males; 85% of impacted canines are palatal to the arch, 8% of patients with impacted canines have bilateral impactions, and there is a small risk (0.35%) of lower canines becoming impacted (Dachi and Howell, 1961; Richardson and McKay, 1982; Ericson and Kurol, 1987).

The aetiology of the impaction is obscure but is probably multifactorial; different theories have been put forward for palatal and buccal impactions (Peck et al., 1994). The maxillary canine, which has the longest path of eruption, is thought to become impacted due to arch length deficiency (Coulter and Richardson, 1997).

Once the impacted canine tooth has been localised, the prognosis of the impacted tooth can be established. Factors affecting its prognosis include patient cooperation, age, general oral health, skeletal variation and the presence of spacing or crowding in the arch. There are six options for treatment: no treatment, interceptive extractions (Figure 4.43), surgical exposure, surgical exposure together with orthodontic alignment, transplantation or extraction (Hunt, 1977; McDonald and Yap, 1986; Ericson and Kurol, 1988b; Sandler et al., 1989; Power and Short, 1993).

The treatment options for surgical exposure fall into three categories: open surgical exposure; open surgical exposure and packing with subsequent bonding of an auxiliary attachment; and closed surgical exposure and bonding of an attachment intraoperatively (Figures 4.44 and 4.45). The first of these method is the most useful when the canine has the correct inclination and will then erupt spontaneously. The

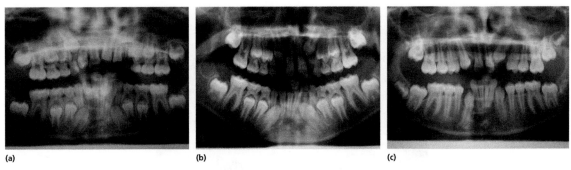

(a)   (b)   (c)

Figure 4.43 Early extraction of teeth whether they are deciduous or permanent can influence the path of eruption of the permanent canines if carried out early enough. These three OPG radiographs were taken in (a) August 2009, (b) October 2010, and (c) October 2012; the improvement in the angulation of the developing teeth can be clearly seen. This intervention has avoided lengthy orthodontic treatment to bring the canines into the dental arch.

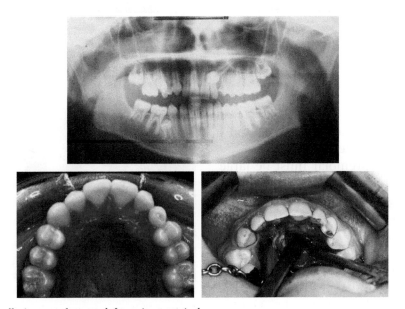

Figure 4.44 Palatally impacted upper left canine; surgical access.

second option is suitable if the tooth is near the surface. Once an attachment is placed, the impacted tooth can then be orthodontically aligned with traction from an appliance. The closed surgical option involves a gold chain being directly bonded to the impacted tooth and the gingival tissues replaced over it (Hunt, 1977). The chain must be very carefully placed as loss of the attachment to the bracket can be very challenging for the orthodontist and patient as a further surgical procedure will be necessary to replace it. However, this is a very effective method for bringing ectopically

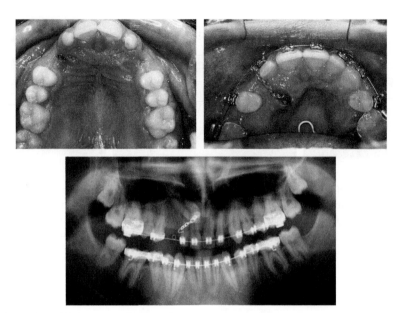

Figure 4.45 Attaching the gold chain to a fixed appliance.

positioned canines into the dental arch and leads to good gingival contour, but it must be remembered that the space between the lateral incisor and premolar must be large enough for the tooth to be accommodated and that pulling the canine into the line of the dental arch takes considerable anchorage. Burden *et al.* (1999) have reported that the failure rate of bonded attachments is about 17% and suggested that the amount of bone removal and type of orthodontic movement needed to align the ectopic canine were more important variables influencing long-term periodontal health.

A modern approach is to reduce appliance time for the patient by attaching the gold chain via an elastic to a temporary anchorage device (TAD) placed in the lower arch. This positioning (Figure 4.46) gives an excellent vector of force to pull the tooth down and avoids the patient having to delay traction until the clinician can

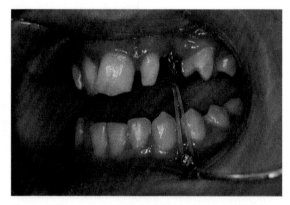

Figure 4.46 A modern approach to provide vertical traction and avoid the long-term use of fixed appliances using a temporary anchorage device (TAD).

place wires in the orthodontic appliance that are stiff enough to support the force of the traction without their distortion. This approach, whilst ideal in terms of reducing the chance of decalcification (in the presence of poor oral hygiene) and poor aes-

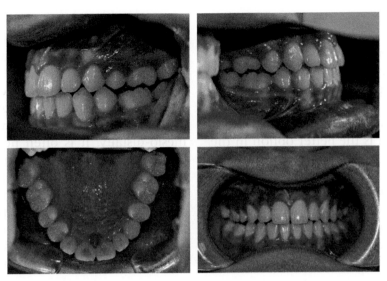

Figure 4.47 Final occlusion following extraction of the upper left maxillary canine. This can be considered to reduce the orthodontic treatment time.

thetics, does demand patient cooperation as the patient is responsible for placing the elastic traction.

To further enhance aesthetics during this treatment it is also possible to leave the primary canine in place and bring the permanent canine slightly palatal to the line of the arch. This may lengthen the treatment time as the permanent tooth is not brought down into the ideal place initially, but does avoid a teenager having a large gap between the incisors and premolars for a considerable length of time. Once the canine has been brought into the mouth, it can be decided if this tooth can be accommodated into the dental arch or whether extraction is necessary.

However, today's restorative advances mean that the extraction of the ectopic canine is a real consideration. A premolar correctly positioned with good buccal root torque to mimic the buccal canine bulge and slightly rotated to hide the palatal cusp can be a very aesthetic alternative. It is even possible to achieve canine guidance in some cases, although group function is the goal (Figure 4.47). When the ectopic canine is a long way from the correct position, it is often worth considering removing it and bringing the first premolar forward. This will often give an excellent cosmetic and functional occlusion.

Missing teeth

Missing upper lateral incisors

Where upper lateral incisors are missing, there is often a dilemma as to whether to close or open the space. Of course, this decision should be based on the malocclusion as a whole as well as the wishes of the patient; however, there are a number of options to consider. There are considerable advantages to having a healthy dentition with no prosthetic placement. If the canine teeth are of good size, shape and colour, they can make an excellent replacement for the lateral incisor with some composite additions and cusp tip trimming. On the other hand, the single tooth implant has also made the management of anterior spacing predictable and effective. The decision as to which is the better option in the long term is often based on the wishes of the patient and the underlying skeletal relationship (Figure 4.48).

While the colour, shape and size of the canine are very important, a decision is commonly made before the canine has erupted. If this is the case, the patient will be making the decision 'blind'. Good photographs of the different options should be used to inform patients as to the aesthetic alternatives.

If implants are contemplated, it is important to ensure there is enough bone in the alveolar area labio-palatally as well as mesio-distally. It is often helpful to allow the upper canine to erupt into the lateral incisor space before retracting it to bring alveolar bone into the area (Figure 4.49). This option also leaves the patient with a large gap as the canine erupts. This can be distressing and must be discussed before treatment commences (Figure 4.50).

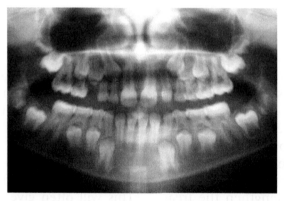

Figure 4.48 Missing upper right lateral incisor.

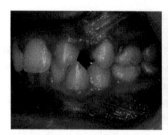 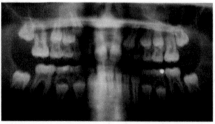

Figure 4.49 Early extraction of the deciduous anterior teeth to guide the permanent canines more easily.

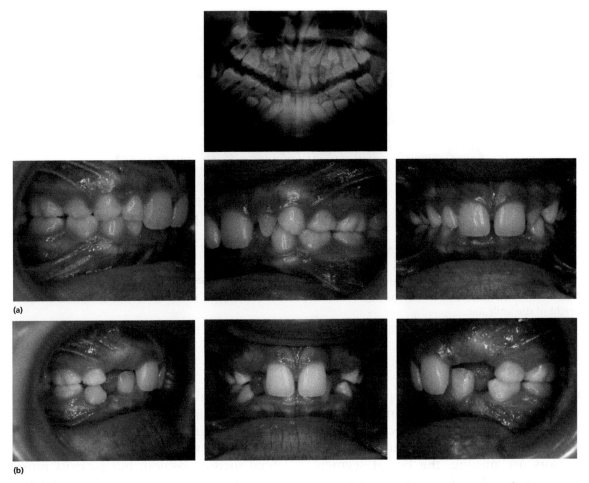

(a)

(b)

Figure 4.50 (a,b) Early extraction of primary teeth guides the second dentition, but may leave unaesthetic spaces during the teenage years. This can be traumatic for the patient.

Closing the anterior space for missing lateral incisors

This option is particularly useful in case of a mild skeletal Class II pattern with an element of crowding, as the space created by the missing lateral incisors can be used to eliminate the crowding or reduce an overjet. In these circumstances, early extraction of the primary lateral incisors or canines can be useful to guide the upper canine teeth into a more mesial position, avoiding the need for long periods of fixed appliance orthodontics. Almost all canines placed in the lateral incisor position will require some form of cosmetic improvement. This will often include the grinding of the incisal tip and the 'squaring off' of the mesial aspect of the canine, making it look more like a lateral incisor tooth. It is particularly important to take account of the upper lip line when deciding on closing an upper anterior space as

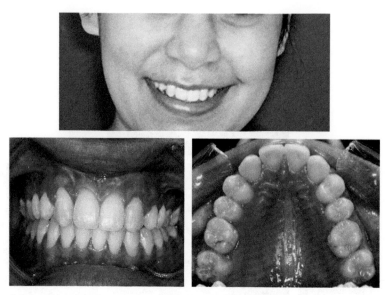

Figure 4.51 The aesthetics of having the upper maxillary canine in the upper lateral incisor space depends on the height of the smile line.

the gingival margin of the upper canine is very much more rounded and narrower than the lateral incisor and can often be unsightly (Figure 4.51). Of course, if lateral incisors are missing, the buccal segment interdigitation is unlikely to be ideal, and it is important to assess the interocclusal relationship and consider some form of interocclusal equilibration to ensure there are no non-working side interferences. Once the upper canines have been brought into the lateral incisor position, the upper first premolars function as if they were canines. In order to improve the aesthetics, it is often a good idea to torque the roots of the upper first premolars buccally to provide a slight canine eminence, and to rotate the premolars mesio-labially so that the palatal cusp is well hidden from direct view. Rotating the premolar mesially also slightly increases the mesio-distal width of

the tooth, which is helpful in terms of the occlusal relationship. With today's excellent restorative materials, it is rare that an upper canine will be unsightly in an upper lateral incisor position, but patients must be warned that they will require life-long minor cosmetic restorative treatment in order to maintain the aesthetics.

Where one lateral incisor is missing or where there is a peg-shaped incisor with a good root, careful assessment of aesthetics needs to be made before deciding whether to keep or lose this tooth. It is often helpful to have the input of a restorative dentist. With unilateral missing lateral incisors, there is of course the option of retaining one lateral incisor and moving the canine into the position of the other or removing the remaining lateral incisor, moving both canines mesially and maintaining symmetry. In these situations, very careful discus-

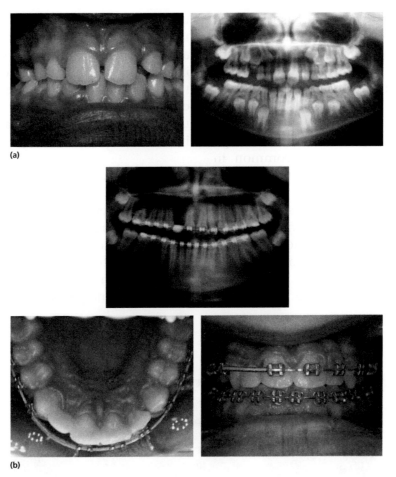

(a)

(b)

Figure 4.52 (a) Preparing space for the replacement of one missing lateral incisor. (b) Using a composite crown form bonded onto an adjacent tooth to keep ideal aesthetics during tooth movement.

sion is required with the patient and restorative dentist to ensure the best aesthetic outcome (Figure 4.52a). The decision as to whether to have an asymmetrical smile but with no missing units, or to open up a space for the unilaterally missing lateral incisor and provide an implant or bridge, is often as much dictated by the malocclusion as the patient's wishes. It is therefore essential that in terms of informed consent, patients have all options explained fully to them (Figure 4.52b).

During treatment, it is important to preserve aesthetics. Bonding a composite crown form to an adjacent tooth preserves the patient's smile and does not interfere with orthodontic tooth movement. As the space opens or closes, the crown form can be modified accordingly.

Opening the anterior space for missing lateral incisors

Opening space for missing lateral incisors or unilaterally missing incisors is of course common in cases where there is intra-arch spacing or a Class III skeletal pattern reduction in overjet (Figure 4.53). Where space opening is the treatment of choice, it is important to ensure that there is at least 7 mm between the roots of the central incisors and canines, to ensure that implant placement is possible if there is enough alveolar bone present. It is common in these circumstances to initially place AERBs until a patient reaches maturity, as the implant (which is in essence anky-losed) will be 'left behind' in a growing patient. When opening space for the provision of a pontic in the upper lateral incisor space, it is very awkward to control the labial palatal position of the root of the upper canines and great care must be taken to ensure that the torque of these teeth is adequate. Group function will be required in terms of the functional occlusion so that the occlusion is not loaded entirely on the canine teeth, which initially is likely to be through the abutment of an anterior lateral incisor resin retained bridge.

Managing space for missing central incisors

When an upper central incisor is missing, it is usually preferable to open the space as the emergence profile of the central incisor with respect to the gingival margin is very different from that of the lateral incisor to the gingival margin. In patients who have

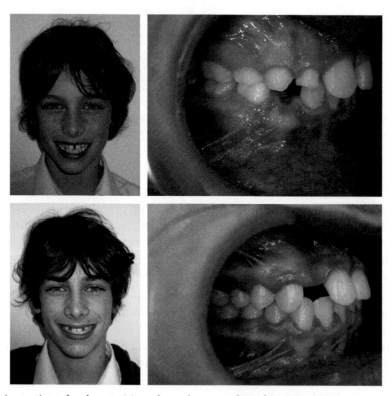

Figure 4.53 Preparing patients for the provision of a replacement lateral incisor.

a low lip line, and particularly a low smile line, moving the lateral incisor into the central incisor position can sometimes be a reasonable solution if the malocclusion allows, but before deciding on this option, careful consideration is required of the anterior aesthetics. In cases of missing central incisors, either due to a supernumerary causing eruption disturbance or a dilaceration or trauma, difficult treatment planning decisions need to be made. Centre-line preservation is essential and treatment planning for a missing central incisor should always involve a restorative dentist as well as an orthodontist. When there has been trauma, there is often loss of the alveolus and this needs to be assessed by CBCT in order to determine whether or not implant placement will be possible in the future. If there is loss of bone, moving a lateral incisor into the position of the central incisor may bring alveolar bone with it and preserve the ridge height. This, as previously stated (Figure 4.23), will compromise the emergence profile of the gingival margin, and full informed consent must be gained from the patient before treatment is started. Often, in order to create enough space to replace the central incisor, a premolar tooth will need to be extracted and careful treatment planning is required whenever healthy teeth are to be extracted following the previous loss of permanent teeth.

With respect to the lower incisor teeth, as the alveolus in this area is often thin and the teeth small, implant placement is difficult or impossible. Where there is loss of a lower incisor, the best treatment option is usually to open the space for the provision of an AERB. Where there is severe crowding or a skeletal Class III pattern, three incisors can be aligned to provide some camouflage for the Class III skeletal

relationship. Each case must be individually assessed before deciding on the treatment options and any plan should be managed by an orthodontist with specialist training.

Missing posterior teeth

When second premolars are missing, assessment of the malocclusion may lead to the decision to extract the second deciduous molars early to allow the first permanent molars to drift forward, thus aiding space closure physiologically. If the malocclusion dictates that the space should be maintained, consideration should be given to interproximal reduction of the second deciduous molar to the size of a permanent second premolar in order that the malocclusion during orthodontic treatment can be treated comprehensively with good buccal segment interdigitation. This tooth can then be left in place until it naturally exfoliates and then immediately replaced with an implant or bridge.

Poor prognosis first permanent molars

The traditional approach to the management of poor prognosis first molars is to consider the malocclusion and carry out either balancing or compensating extractions to manage the loss of the affected tooth. It is generally accepted that the best timing of the extraction of the first molars is once the furcation of the second molars can be identified radiographically. However, there is no well-documented evidence to support this and with modern orthodontic appliances, it is now more reasonable to assess the malocclusion as a whole and the prognosis of each individual tooth, rather than condemning teeth with a good prognosis to extraction purely to provide a symmetrical occlusion. With modern orthodontic appliances and the use of

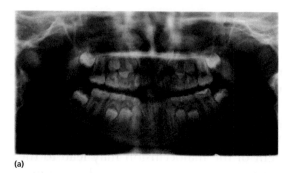 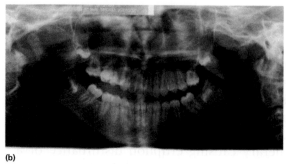

(a)   (b)

Figure 4.54 (a) Pre- and (b) post-extraction of the first permanent molars showing good replacement by second molars.

TADs, the vertical development of teeth can be stabilised during treatment and therefore individual first molars can be extracted without the need to extract the opposing teeth (Figure 4.54). In order to manage crowding, the decision either to keep first molars as a space maintainer or lose them early in order to provide space for the mesial drift of second molars can be an important one, as it will affect the complexity of the orthodontic treatment in the long term. Where there is crowding in the upper arch and an overjet, maintaining the upper first molars until the second molars have erupted so that a palatal arch can be placed on them, can provide space for the distilisation of buccal segments and eventual reduction of the overjet. Often, extracting lower first molars early to allow the lower second molars to drift mesially reduces the amount of space closure required and therefore the likelihood of retroclination of the lower labial segment.

No simple rules can be provided for the complex decision to extract poor prognosis first molars; however, assessment by a specialist orthodontist is always advised and early planning is in the patient's best interest.

References

Baccetti T, Leonardi M, Armi P. (2008) A randomized clinical study of two interceptive approaches to palatally displaced canines. Eur J Orthod. 30(4): 381–385.

Bailey LJ, Proffit WR, White R Jr. (1999) Assessment of patients for orthognathic surgery. Semin Orthod. 5(4): 209–222.

Brennan MM, Gianelly AA. (2000) The use of the lingual arch in the mixed dentition to resolve incisor crowding. Am J Orthod Dentofacial Orthop. 117(1): 81–85.

Burden DJ, Mullally BH, Robinson SN. (1999) Palatally ectopic canines: closed eruption versus open eruption. Am J Orthod Dentofacial Orthop. 115(6): 640–644.

Collett AR. (2000) Conservative management of lower second premolar impaction. Aust Dent J. 45(4): 279–281.

Coulter J, Richardson A. (1997) Normal eruption of the maxillary canine quantified in three dimensions. Eur J Orthod. 19(2): 171–183.

Czochrowska EM, Skaare AB, Stenvik A, Zachrisson BU. (2003) Outcome of orthodontic space closure with a missing maxillary central incisor. Am J Orthod Dentofacial Orthop. 123(6): 597–603.

Dachi SF, Howell FV. (1961) A survey of 3,874 routine full-month radiographs. II. A study of impacted teeth. Oral Surg Oral Med Oral Pathol. 14: 1165–1169.

DiBiase DD. (1968–1969) Midline supernumeraries and eruption of maxillary central incisors. Trans BSSO: 83–88.

Ericson S, Kurol J. (1987) Radiographic examination of ectopically erupting maxillary canines. Am J Orthod Dentofacial Orthop. 91(6): 483–492.

Ericson S, Kurol J. (1988a) Early treatment of palatally erupting maxillary canines by extraction of the primary canines. Eur J Orthod. 10: 283–295.

Ericson S, Kurol J. (1988b) Resorption of maxillary lateral incisors caused by ectopic eruption of the canines. A clinical and radiographic analysis of predisposing factors. Am J Orthod Dentofacial Orthop. 94(6): 503–513.

Fränkel R. (1966) The theoretical concept underlying the treatment with function correctors. Rep Congr Eur Orthod Soc. 42, 233–254.

Hunt NP. (1977) Direct traction applied to unerupted teeth using the acid-etch technique. Br J Orthod. 4(4): 211–212.

Mason C, Azam N, Holt RD, Rule DC. (2000) A retrospective study of unerupted maxillary incisors associated with supernumerary teeth. Br J Oral Maxillofac Surg. 38(1): 62–65.

McDonald F, Yap WL. (1986) The surgical exposure and application of direct traction of unerupted teeth. Am J Orthod. 89(4): 331–340.

Mitchell L. (2000) An Introduction to Orthodontics, 2nd edn. Oxford University Press, Oxford.

Ngan P, Alkire RG, Fields H Jr. (2000) Management of space problems in the primary and mixed dentitions. J Am Dent Assoc. 131(1): 16, 18.

O'Brien K, Macfarlane T, Wright J, et al. (2009) Early treatment for Class II Division 1 malocclusion with the Twin-block appliance: a multi-center, randomized, controlled trial. Am J Orthod Dentofacial Orthop. 135(5): 580–585.

Mistry P, Moles DR, O'Neill J, Noar J. (2010) The occlusal effects of digit sucking habits amongst school children in Northamptonshire (UK). J Orthod. 37: 87–92.

Patel A. (2008) Digit sucking in children resident in Kettering (UK). J Orthod. 35: 255–261.

Peck S, Peck L, Kataja M. (1994) The palatally displaced canine as a dental anomaly of genetic origin. Angle Orthod. 64(4): 249–256.

Popovich F. (1966) The prevalence of sucking habit and its relationship to oral malformations. Applied Ther. 8: 689–691.

Power SM, Short MB. (1993) An investigation into the response of palatally displaced canines to the removal of deciduous canines and an assessment of factors contributing to favourable eruption. Br J Orthod. 20(3): 215–223.

Richardson A, McKay C. (1982) Delayed eruption of maxillary canine teeth. Part I. Aetiology and diagnosis. Proc Br Paedod Soc. 12: 15–25.

Sandler PJ, Meghji S, Murray AM, et al. (1989) Magnets and orthodontics. Br J Orthod. 16(4): 243–249.

Tulloch JF, Phillips C, Proffit WR. (1998) Benefit of early Class II treatment: progress report of a two-phase randomized clinical trial. Am J Orthod Dentofacial Orthop. 113(1): 62–72.

Vig PS, Vig KW. (1986) Hybrid appliances: a component approach to dentofacial orthopedics. Am J Orthod Dentofacial Orthop. 90(4): 273–285.

Warren J, Slayton R, Yonezu T, Bishara S, Levy S, Kanellis M. (2005). Effects of nonnutritive sucking habits on occlusal characteristics in the mixed dentition. Pediatr Dent. 27: 445–450.

Witsenberg B, Boering G. (1981) Eruption of impacted permanent incisors after removal of supernumerary teeth. Int J Oral Surg. 10: 423–431.

Zablocki HL, McNamara JA Jr, Franchi L, Baccetti T. (2008) Effect of the transpalatal arch during extraction treatment. Am J Orthod Dentofacial Orthop. 133(6): 852–860.

Index

Note: Page entries in *italics* indicate photos.

Acid-etched retained bridges, 45, 70, 71
Activators, 54
AERBs. *See* Acid-etched retained bridges
Aesthetics. *See* Dental aesthetics; Facial aesthetics
Alignment, 1
Alveolar bone preservation
  bringing teeth into line of dental arch and, 42, *44*
  megadont tooth management and, 47
Ankylosis, fused or geminated teeth and, 47
Anterior crossbites
  causing forward displacement of lower central incisors, 35
  early treatment of, reasons for, 35
  extractions and, 35, *36*
  posterior coverage and correction of, *36*
  showing potential damage involving tooth wear and periodontal involvement, 35
  simple removable appliances in treatment for, *36*
  of upper right central incisor, 35
Anterior occlusal radiographs, 15
Anteroposterior (A-P) plane, clinical assessment of, 9, *10*
Anteroposterior (A-P) skeletal relationship, clinical assessment of, 9, *10*
Appliance therapy
  behavioral management and, 58
  thumb/digit sucking and, 30, *30*
Appliance time, reducing, 64
Appliances. *See also* Functional appliances; Orthodontic appliances
  care of, 57
  first fit and, 55, 57
  fixed, for closing anterior incisor spacing, *34*
  posterior expansion and, 37
  removable, for anterior crossbites, *36*
  younger patient and compliance with, 51
Arch expansion
  upper, with removable appliance to eliminate unilateral crossbite, *38*
  views of, 37
Asymmetries
  mandibular displacements as cause of, *12*
  mild transverse, 11
Attractive smiles, importance of, 9
Autotransplantation, of crowded premolars, considerations with, 42

Balance, facial aesthetics and, 9
Band and loop space maintainers, submerging lower left second deciduous molar and, 45–46, *46*
Behavioral management, appliance therapy and, 58
Bite planes, anterior crossbites and, 35
Bite registration, overbite and, 55
Bonded attachments, failure rate of, 64
Boys, peak height velocity in, 5
Buccal crossbites, 33

Calvarium, growth of, 5
Canines
  as 'cornerstone' of arch, 62
  ectopic, extraction of, 65
  impacted
    incidence of, 62
    palatally, upper left and surgical access, *63*
  permanent, early extractions and path of eruption of, *63*
  primary, extraction of, 39
    crowding and, 32, *32*
    preventing center-line shift and, 32
Caries, 14
CBCT. *See* Cone-beam computed tomography
Center-line shift, preventing, early extraction of primary canines and, 32
Central incisors
  geminated, 47
  large upper, managing, *48*
  managing space for, 70–71
  mesiodens supernumeraries preventing eruption of, *43*
  tuberculate supernumeraries preventing eruption of, *42*
  unerupted, *42*, 45
Cephalometric evaluation, 16–17
Chincup therapy, 59, *60*, *61*
Chondrocranium, 2
Clark Twin Block, *54*
Class I malocclusions, 50
Class I molar relationship, stable, leeway space and, 50
Class I relationship, maxilla position relative to mandible and, 9
Class II malocclusions, treatment option for, 51
Class II sagittal problems. *See* Sagittal problems: Class II
Class III malocclusions, treatment options for, 59
Class III sagittal problems. *See* Sagittal problems: Class III
Class III skeletal pattern, managing space for missing central incisors and, 70

Interceptive Orthodontics: A Practical Guide to Occlusal Management, First Edition. Joseph Noar.
© 2014 John Wiley & Sons, Ltd. Published 2014 by John Wiley & Sons, Ltd.

Class III traction elastics, 59
Clinical assessment
    of A-P skeletal relationship, *10*
    of facial symmetry, 11, *12*
    of lower anterior face height, *11*
    of maxillary mandibular angle, *11*
    of overjet, 12, *12*
    tools, *10*
Closed surgical exposure, bonding of attachment
        intraoperatively, 62, 63
Cognitive behavioral management, thumb/digit sucking and, 30
Compliance with appliances
    better facial balance and reinforcement of, 53
    functional appliances and, 57–58
    Quadhelix appliances and eliminating need for, *38*
    younger patients and, 51
Condylar cartilage, traditional view of, 3
Cone-beam computed tomography, 17–18
    developmental anomalies detected with, *21*, 21–22
    impacted/ectopic teeth detected with, 18
    managing space for missing central incisors and assessment
        with, 71
    root fracture detected with, *22, 23*
    root resorption association with impacted teeth detected
        with, 18–19, *19*
    supernumerary teeth detected with, 19, *20*, 21
    tooth position assessed with, 42
    uses for, 17
    volumetric data set obtained with, 18
Cortical drift principle, 4
Cranial base, growth of, 2
Craniofacial growth and development, 4–5
    cephalometric evaluation of, 16
    components in, 2
    genetics and, 5
Craniofacial skeleton, growth and development of, 2
Crossbites
    anterior, 35, *35, 36*
    appliance wear and, 30
    posterior, 37–38
        correcting, 33
    unilateral, upper arch expansion with removable appliance for
        elimination of, *38*
Crowding, 52, 61
    assessing on OPG radiographs, 16
    closing anterior space for missing lateral incisors and, 64
    large upper central incisors (megadont teeth) and, *48*
    leeway space and, 50
    managing space for missing central incisors and, 68
    of permanent lateral incisors, 32–34
    poor prognosis first molars and, 71
    of primary canines, before and after extraction, 32, *32*
    severe, OPG radiographs showing management of with
        interceptive extractions, *42*
    study casts and assessment of, 23
    submerging deciduous second molars and, 45, *46*
Crown form, composite, bonding to adjacent tooth, 69
Cybernetic model of growth regulation, 5

Deciduous extractions
    anterior crossbites and, 35
    early, crowding and premise behind, 33
Deciduous second molars, submerging, 46–47

Delayed eruption, supernumerary teeth and, 42
Dental aesthetics. *See also* Facial aesthetics
    age considerations and need for, 26
    life-long cosmetic restorative treatment and, 68
Dental arch, 9
    non-appliance guiding of adult teeth into line of, 34
    shape of, 1
    thumb/finger sucking and distortion of, 29
Dental attractiveness, goals in aiming for, 1
Dental history, 9
Dental mirrors, *10*
Dental panoramic tomograms
    localizing impacted teeth with, 18
    supernumerary tooth associated with upper left central incisor
        in, *20*
Dental tissue, quality and morphology of, 1
Dental wax, postured position for functional appliance and, 57
Dentition position, racial and sexual differences in, 9
Development, defined, 2
Developmental anomalies, CBCT and detection of, *21*, 21–22
Digit sucking, 29–30
    asymmetric open bite due to, *29*
    preventing, with fixed thumb guard, *30*
Digital photography, 24
Dilaceration of root, unerupted tooth and, 42
Displacement principle, 4
DPTs. *See* Dental panoramic tomograms

Early interceptive treatment, premise behind, 1
Eating, large upper labial frenum and effect on, 48
Ectopic teeth, 62–65. *See also* Impacted teeth
    CBCT and detection of, 18
    incidence of, 62
    occlusal guidance and, 39
    severely, complex orthodontic treatment for, *44*
Ectopically positioned teeth
    early assessment and, 15
    managing, methods of, 42
Enamel hypoplasias, 14
Endochondral ossification, 2
Epiphyseal plate, 3
Expansion, early, as effective environment for permanent tooth
        development, 33
Expansion appliances, 30
Extractions
    anterior crossbites and, 35, 36
    assessing crowding on OPG radiographs and, 16
    early
        of deciduous anterior teeth, to guide permanent canines
            more easily, 63
        path of eruption of permanent canines and, 61
        of primary teeth and unaesthetic spaces seen during teenage
            years, 67
    early treatment of Class II sagittal problems combined
        with, 52
    of ectopic canines, 65
    good oral hygiene and, 33
    interceptive
        crowding and, 33
        of impacted teeth, 63
        OPG radiographs showing management of severe crowding
            with, *41*
    poor prognosis first permanent molars and, 71

of premolars, managing space for missing central incisors and, 71

of primary canines, 62

to prevent center-line shift, 32

understanding consequences of crowding for patient and, 33

of second deciduous molars, 45, 71

serial, 39, *40–41*

of upper left maxillary canine, final occlusion after, *65*

Extraoral photographs, *25*

Face, growth patterns of, 4

Facemasks, 59

Facial aesthetics

factors related to, 9

good, description of, 11

Facial attractiveness, importance of, 9

Facial form

assessment of, 11–12

overall impression of, 9

Facial growth, directions of, *2*

Facial profile, early treatment of Class II sagittal problems and, 52

Facial proportions, vertical, assessing, 10–11

Facial skeleton

growth fields and, 3–4

growth of, 5

Facial sutures, adaptive growth and, 3

Finger sucking. *See* Digit sucking; Thumb/finger sucking

Finger/thumb splints, 30

Fixed appliance treatment, decline in, 39

Fixed appliances, 54, 59

Class III malocclusion treated with, *60, 61*

for closing anterior incisor spacing, *34*

gold chain attached to, 62, *62*

leeway space management and, 50

Fixed thumb guard, 30, *30*

Food traps, submerging lower left second deciduous molar and, 45, *46*

Fracture and luxation, of anterior teeth, *52*

Fränkel appliances, 54

Fränkel II functional regulator (FRII), 55

Frankfort plane, 10

Functional appliances

bite registration and, 55

compliance and, 53

day-to-day management of, 57

first fit for, 55, 57

maintaining any changes and, 53

parental involvement and, 55

poor compliance and, 57

serial extraction combined with, 39

struggling child and, 58

tooth movement pattern and, 53

types and designs for, *54,* 54–55

Functional matrix theory, 5

Functional regulator II appliance, *54,* 55

Fused teeth

CBCT showing extent of root and crown contact, 22, *22*

planning for, 47

Geminated teeth

CBCT and assessment of, 22

central incisor, 47

planning for, 47

General dental practitioners (GDPs), referrals by, 1

General environmental influences, skeletal morphogenesis and, 5

General epigenetic factors, skeletal morphogenesis and, 5

Genetic factors, growth and, 5, *6*

Gingival contour, 1

Gingival loss, deep bite and, 13

Gingival margin, managing space for missing central incisors and, 70–71

Girls, peak height velocity in, 5

Glass Ionomer cement, Quadhelix appliance and use of, 37

Gold chain

attaching to fixed appliance, *64*

attaching via an elastic to temporary anchorage device, 64, *64*

bonding to impacted tooth, 63

bonding to unerupted tooth, 42

Growth

of cranial base, 2

defined, 2

of mandible, 3–4

mechanisms of, 2

of mid-face, 3

of nasomaxillary complex, 4

what we know about, 1–5

Growth pattern, 2, 4

Growth rate, 2, 4–5

Growth regulating mechanism, 2, 5

Harmony, facial aesthetics and, 9

Head posture, overall impression of, 9

Headgear

protraction, treatment of Class III malocclusion with, *60, 61*

serial extraction combined with, 39

Height velocity, peak, in girls and boys, 5

Heredity, growth and, 5

Hybrid appliances, 54

Hypodontia, 15, 37

Impacted incisors, managing: the treatment sequence, *43*

Impacted teeth, 62–65

CBCT and detection of, 18

root resorption associated with, 18–19, *19*

defined, 62

establishing prognosis for, 62

treatment options for, 62

surgical exposure, categories, 62–64

Implants, 45, 66, 68, 71

Incisor spacing, anterior, closing with use of fixed appliances, *34*

Incisors

central

geminated, 47

mesiodens supernumeraries preventing eruption of, *43*

tuberculate supernumeraries preventing eruption of, *42*

unerupted, 42, 45

clinical assessment of

at about age 7, 62

overjet and, 12–13, *13*

functional appliance and changes in, 57

fusion of, periapical radiograph showing, 22

impacted, 62

managing: the treatment sequence, *43*

large upper central, *48*

Incisors (*cont'd*)
  lateral
    moved into central incisor position, 45, *45*
    preparing patients for provision of replacement, *70*
    replacement of one missing, *69*
  lip traps and, *49*
  lower central, anterior crossbite causing forward displacement
    of, *35*
  missing
    central, managing space for, 70–71
    lateral, closing anterior space for, 67–69, *69*
    lateral, opening anterior space for, 69–70
    upper lateral, 65–66
    upper right, *66*
  permanent lateral, crowding of, 32–34
  proclination of upper, risk of trauma and, *51*
  prominent, retroclination of, *53*
  upper, normal size of, *47*
  upper right central, anterior crossbite of, *35*
Informed consent
  managing space for missing central incisors and, 71
  retainer wear and, 37
  unilateral missing lateral incisors and, 67
Interceptive extractions
  crowding and advantages with, 33
  OPG radiographs showing management of severe crowding
    with, 41
Interocclusal equilibration, closing anterior space for missing
    lateral incisors and, 65
Intramembranous ossification, 2
Intraoral anchorage arches, leeway space and use of, 50, *50*
Intraoral photographs, *25*
Intraoral rulers, overjet and overbite measured with, 12,
    12
Intrinsic genetic factors, skeletal morphogenesis and, 5
Intrusive activators, 54

Jaws, 9
  cephalometric evaluation of position of, 16
  growth and development of, 2–4

Labial frenum, prominent, removal of, 48–49
Large teeth, managing, 47, *48*
Lateral cephalograms, 18
Lateral cephalographs and analysis, 16, *17*
Lateral incisors
  fused or geminated teeth and, 47
  missing
    opening anterior space for, 69–70
    replacement of, *69*
    upper, 65–66
  moving into central incisor space, 45, *45*
  permanent, crowding of, 32–34
  replacement, preparing patients for provision of, *70*
Leeway space
  defined, 50
  intraoral anchorage arches and, 50
  preserving, with palatal and lingual arches, 50–51, *51*
Lingual arch
  preserving leeway space with, 50, *50*
  for stabilizing molar position and arch length after loss of
    primary second molar, 46
  using to provide point of traction, *63*

Lip apart posture at rest, 13, *13*
Lip line
  managing space for missing central incisors and, 67
  upper, closing upper anterior space and, 65
Lip traps, *13*
  causing proclination of upper central incisors and retroclination
    of lower incisors, *49*
  causing proclination of upper right central incisor, *49*
  early treatment of, 49
  eliminating, 53
Local environmental influences, skeletal morphogenesis
    and, 5
Local epigenetic factors, skeletal morphogenesis and, 5
Lower anterior face height, clinical assessment of, *11*

Malocclusions. *See also* Sagittal problems: Class II
  Class II, treatment options for, 51–55
  Class III, *59*
  fused or geminated teeth and, 47
  thumb/finger sucking and, 29
Mandible
  chincup and restraint of, 59
  growth of, 3–4
    Class III patients and, 59
  orthodontic change and, 24
  rough position of maxilla relative to, 9
Mandibular condyle, cartilage of, 3
Mandibular displacement, due to crossbites with
    displacements, *12*
Mandibular rotations, cephalometric evaluation of, 16
Mastication muscles, functional appliances and, 54
Maxilla
  Class III patients and growth of, 59
  facemasks and protraction of, 59
  orthodontic change and, 24
  rough position of, relative to mandible, 9
Maxillary arch expansion, for child *vs.* for adult, 37
Maxillary canine, impaction of, 62
Maxillary complex, direction of growth of, 4
Maxillary incisors, unerupted supernumerary teeth and impaction
    of, 19
Maxillary mandibular angle, clinical assessment of, *11*
Median diastema, large upper labial fraenum and, 48
Median opening activator, *54*, 55
Medical history, 9
Megadont teeth
  managing, 47, *48*
  orthodontic tooth movement and restorative management
    of, *48*
Mesiodens supernumeraries, preventing eruption of central
    incisors, 43
Mid-face, growth of, 3
Missing teeth, 65–72
  closing anterior space for missing lateral incisors,
    67–69
  managing space for missing central incisors, 70–71
  missing posterior teeth, 71–72
  missing upper lateral incisors, 65–66
  missing upper right lateral incisor, 66
  opening anterior space for missing lateral incisors,
    69–70
  poor prognosis first permanent molars, 71
MM angle, assessing, 10–11

Molars
  deciduous second, submerging, 45–46
  first permanent
    poor prognosis, 71
    pre- and post-extraction of, showing good replacement by
        second molars, *72*
  third, impacted, 62

Nail paint, 30
Nasal septal cartilage, growth of, 3
Nasomaxillary complex, growth of, 4
Non-compliance, clearly stating downsides of, 57

OB. *See* Overbite
Occlusal guidance, modern, 39
Occlusal radiographs, 18
Odontomes, 62
OJ. *See* Overjet
Open bite
  anterior, forward tongue position, *13*
  asymmetric, due to digit sucking, *29*
Open surgical exposure, packing with subsequent bonding of
    auxiliary attachment and, 62
OPG radiographs. *See* Orthopantogram (OPG) radiographs
Oral hygiene, 13, 14, 64
  acid-etched retained bridges and, 45
  extractions and, 34
Orthodontic alignment with surgical exposure, ectopic/impacted
    teeth and, 62
Orthodontic appliances
  orthodontic change and, 24
  patients who do well and not so well with, 26
Orthodontic change, scope of, 24, 26
Orthodontic traction, impacted teeth and, 18, 19
Orthodontic treatment
  planning and, 38
  reasons for, 26
  success *vs.* failure of, 26
  timing of, 26
Orthognathic surgery, Class III sagittal problems and, 59
Orthopantogram (OPG) radiographs, 15, 34, 62
  crowding assessed with, 16
  for identifying maxillary canine position using vertical
      parallax, *15*
  posterior expansion and assessment with, 37
  showing management of severe crowding with interceptive
      extractions along, *41*
  showing path of eruption of permanent canines after early
      extractions, *63*
  simple assessment of space requirements with, *15*
  submerging deciduous second molars and, 45
  unerupted central incisor assessed with, 42
Overbite
  appliance wear and, 30
  assessment of, 12
  bite registration and, 55
  soft tissue damage and, 13
  study casts and, 23
Overjet
  appliance wear and, 30
  clinical assessment of, 12, *12*
  functional appliance and reduction in, 58
  functional regulator II appliance and, 55

increased, treatment sequence for management of, *52–53, 56*
trauma risk and, 13
trauma to incisors and, 52

Palatal arches, preserving leeway space with, 50, *50*
Parallax. *See* Vertical parallax
Parental involvement, importance of, 57–58
Patient education, photography and, 24
Periapical views, localizing impacted teeth in, 18
Periodontal disease, 14
Periosteum, as osteogenic zone, 4
Permanent teeth, comprehensive treatment and presence of, 26
Photographs, 24, *25*
  extraoral, *25*
  intraoral, *25*
Physical growth status of child, assessing, 9
Plaque indexes, 14
Plaster study casts, space analysis on, *24*
Poor prognosis first permanent molars, management of, 68–69
Posterior crossbites, 37–38
Posterior teeth, missing, 71–72
Premolars
  first
    erupted and ready for extraction, *40*
    extraction of, 39
    rotating, and mesio-distal width of tooth, 68
  second
    erupting and ready for alignment if required, *40*
    impacted, 62
    impacted, submerging lower right second deciduous molar
        and, *46*
    missing, 71
Primary teeth
  early extraction of, 15
  and unaesthetic spaces seen during teenage years, *67*
Protraction headgear, 59, *60, 61*
Pubertal growth spurt, 5, 26, 51

Quadhelix appliances
  eliminating need for patient compliance with, *38*
  for expanding upper dental arch and correcting lateral arch
      dimensions, *31*
  Glass Ionomer cement and use of, 37
  posterior expansion and, 37, *38*
  uses for, 30

Radiographs, 15. *See also* Orthopantogram (OPG) radiographs
Relocation principle, 4
Remodelling principle, 4
Removable appliances, 54
  for applying traction, *64*
  behavioral management and, 58
Respect, building, 57
Retainer wear, child and commitment to, 37
Retainers, cephalometric evaluation and, 16–17
Root fracture, CBCT and detection of, 22, 23
Root resorption, impacted teeth and, CBCT detection of, 18–19,
    19
Ruler, *10*

Sagittal problems: Class II, 51–59
  day-to-day management, 57
  first fit, 55, 57

Sagittal problems: Class II (*cont'd*)
  functional appliance designs for, *54*
  functional bite registration, 55
  increased overjet, treatment sequence for, *52–53, 56*
  involving the parents, 58
  objections to early treatment for, 51
  poor compliance, dealing with, 57–58
  proclamation of upper incisors increases risk of trauma, *51*
  research on, 51
  result of fall, fracture and luxation of anterior teeth, *51*
  struggling child, 58
Sagittal problems: Class III, 59, *60, 61*
Sagittal treatment, looking at more than growth evidence for, 51
Salivation, appliances and effect on, 57
Second molars, deciduous, submerging, 45–46, *46*
Self-esteem
  early treatment of Class II sagittal problems and, 54
  poor aesthetics and effect on child, 32
Serial extractions
  combined with sagittal correction with headgear or functional appliances, 39
  first premolars erupted and ready for extraction, *40*
  as modern approach, 39
  occlusal management with interceptive extractions and, 39
  second premolars erupting, ready for alignment if required, *40*
  six months after primary canine extraction, *40*
  start of, *40*
Skeletal age, estimating, 5
Skeletal discrepancy, lip traps and, 49
Skeletal morphogenesis, factors involved in, 5
Smile line, 1
  importance of, 9
  managing space for missing central incisors and, 67
  upper maxillary canine in upper lateral incisor space and height of, 67–68, *68*
Somatic tissues, growth rate for, 5
Space maintainers, submerging lower left second deciduous molar and, 45–46
Speech, appliances and effects on, 57
Stability, predicting, cephalometric analysis never used for, 17
Standard occlusal radiograph, 15
Stature, growth in, 5
Struggling child, goals and, 58
Study models or casts, 23, *24*
Supernumerary teeth, 37, 62
  CBCT and detection of, 19, *20, 21*
  delayed eruption and, 42
Surgical exposure
  impacted teeth and, 62–64
  orthodontic alignment with, 61
  treatment options for, categories of, 61–62
Sutural Theory, 3

Symmetry, 1
  clinical assessment of, 11, *12*
  facial aesthetics and, 9, 11
Synchondrosal cartilage, 3

TAD. *See* Temporary anchorage device
Talon cusp, CBCT imaging at different heights, demonstrating degree of extension of pulpal tissue into, *21*
Teasing at school
  poor aesthetics and, 32
  timing of treatment and, 26
  treating Class II sagittal problems and reduction in, 52
Temporary anchorage device
  gold chain attached via an elastic to, 64, *64*
  poor prognosis permanent molars and, 71
Temporomandibular joint (TMJ) function
  anterior crossbites and, 34
  assessing, 14
Third molars, impacted, 62
3 month-6 month rule, poor compliance and, 57–58
Thumb/finger sucking, *29*, 29–30
Thumb guard
  clinical effects of: start, 3 months, 6 months, 9 months, *31*
  fixed, to prevent digit sucking, 30, *30*
Timing of treatment, 26
TMJ function. *See* Temporomandibular joint (TMJ) function
Tongue thrusts, 13, *13*
Tooth brushing, large upper labial frenum and, 48
Tooth inclination, study casts and assessment of, 23
Tooth movement pattern, functional appliances and, 53
Tooth reduction, 48
Traction elastics, Class III, 59
Transplantation, impacted teeth, 61
Trauma
  to incisors, overjets and, 51
  to large upper labial frenum, 48
Treatment. *See* Orthodontic treatment
Tuberculate supernumeraries, preventing eruption of central incisors, *42*

Unilateral crossbite, eliminating, upper arch expansion with removable appliance for, *38*

"V" principle, 4
Vertical parallax, using with OPG radiograph to identify maxillary canine position, 15, *15*
Vertical plane, assessment of, 10–11
Voxels, 18

Wax impressions, postured position for functional appliance and, 55, *57*
Wear time, appliances and, 57

Printed and bound by CPI Group (UK) Ltd, Croydon, CR0 4YY

27/10/2024

14580288-0005